"UNLOCK THE SECRETS OF TRANSFORMATION, BALANCE, AND INNER POWER"

THROUGH THE 5-4-3-2-1 METHOD

SHIVA

THE 5 SACRED STEPS TO SUCCESS AND SERENITY

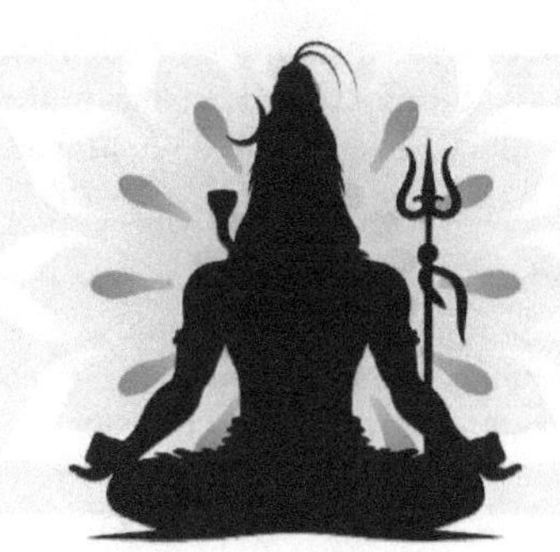

A YOGA AND MEDITATION TECHNIQUE

VAIBHAVI HARIDAS

With Foreward by Swami Atmavidyananda Giri

First Edition

Feb 25, 2025

Book production and publishing – Vaibhavi Haridas and Ethnik Publications

SHIVA

The 5 sacred steps to success and serenity

Author

VAIBHAVI HARIDAS

With Foreword by Swami Atmavidyananda Giri of Kriya Yoga

First edition released on the auspicious occasion of Mahashivratri
Feb 25, 2025

IN MEMORY OF MY GRANDPARENTS

Your wisdom, love, and blessings continue to guide me on this path.

Sankarrao Agwan (27 July 1922 – 18 March 1986)

Vasudeo Joshi (5 January 1924 – 28 September 2014)

Nalini Agwan (Sudha Darwhekar) (19 March 1929 – 23 December 2020)

Nirmala Joshi (Malti Gadre) (18 February 1932 – 22 January 2023)

DEDICATED TO

My Pillars of Strength and Unwavering Support

Vijay Agwan and Medha Agwan– My parents for giving me life, a strong foundation, and the courage to walk my own path.

Aniketa Agwan– My soul sister, my source of strength, and the one who set me on the path of yoga teacher training.

Harshal Haridas– My husband, my heart, my home, my greatest joy.

Arya Haridas and Atharva Haridas – My children, my inspiration, my teachers, my most cherished blessings.

Suresh Haridas and Suhasini Haridas, and Shital Pandit – My in-laws for shaping the man who walks beside me with love, wisdom, and values.

SPECIAL THANKS

Swami Atmavidyanand Giri of Kriya Yoga for your profound service spirit and offering of live yoga philosophy topics on Arva Yoga platform. Your guidance and tremendous support and words of encouragement for this initiative are a blessing in itself.

GRATITUDE

My extended family, friends, yoga students, editors, mentors, and gurus—each of you has played a role in shaping my journey, helping me discover my true self.

And to all the souls who came before me, and all those who will come after—

To the seekers, the questioners, the ones who dare to ask: "Who am I?"

चिदानन्दरूपः शिवोऽहम् शिवोऽहम्

(I am the form of pure consciousness and bliss. I am Shiva, I am Shiva.)

NOTE TO READERS

For as long as I can remember, I have felt a deep, unshakable connection to Lord Shiva. Each time I have been blessed to visit Kedarnath Temple, an overwhelming sense of divinity has enveloped me—an experience beyond words, a presence that transcends time and space. This book is titled SHIVA as a tribute to that sacred connection, but more importantly, to honor the omnipresence of Lord Shiva in every living and non-living entity in the universe. You can just as easily replace SHIVA with any name of that divine power that shines in all of us- God, Allah, Jesus Christ, Shree Krishna, Devi, Light, Truth, Origin and countless more names that exist.

My personal and professional stories are for another time and space. This book, however, is my offering—a concise yet powerful guide that distills the essence of a proprietary technique I have developed over years of dedicated yoga and meditation practice, primarily geared toward a busy professional. Over the past six years, I have had the privilege of guiding countless students—both beginners and seasoned practitioners—through structured, transformative yoga sessions. And in this journey as a yoga teacher, I have developed a proprietary framework for each practice that I am sharing with the world with this book. The SHIVA Technique and 5-4-3-2-1 Method offer a unique, holistic approach to integrating physical asanas and meditative practices in a way that maximizes benefits while seamlessly fitting into the demanding lives of modern professionals. If you are familiar with yoga and meditation but struggle with consistency, lack structure, or are seeking a reliable daily routine—this book is for you.

If you believe that yoga and meditation might slow down your professional growth, think again! These techniques are designed to sharpen the mind, strengthen the body, and enhance focus—allowing you to achieve external professional success with greater ease and clarity. Whether you're navigating high-pressure environments, ethical dilemmas, or complex workplace dynamics, this practice empowers you to make decisions from a place of calm and confidence.

This book is also for those who feel adrift in life—whether you feel trapped in a role that seems small or been recently laid off or you are an overworked parent who has no time for your own self-care. Start small. Implement this technique. Find clarity, align with your true purpose, and begin living fully and intentionally.

Whether you choose to read this book cover to cover, read any one chapter for some insights or dive straight into the methodology in the appendix for a structured day-by-day practice guide, my hope is that it serves as a compass on your journey to balance, strength, and inner peace.

INTRODUCTION TO THIS BOOK

This book is designed as a comprehensive yet practical guide to help you integrate yoga, meditation, and the timeless wisdom of Lord Shiva into your daily life. It is divided into three parts—each focusing on a distinct aspect of the philosophical teachings, structured methodology, and practical application—along with an appendix for further reference.

Who Is This Book For?

Whether you are a seasoned yoga practitioner, a curious beginner, or someone simply seeking balance, clarity, and strength, this book is for you. You will find immense value in its teachings if:

- You are drawn to the wisdom of Lord Shiva and want to explore his significance beyond mythology—as a symbol of transformation, resilience, and inner mastery.
- You wish to deepen your yoga and meditation practice by incorporating structure, intention, and a holistic approach.
- You are looking to develop a sustainable daily yoga routine that fits seamlessly into your modern, fast-paced life.
- You are a busy professional navigating the corporate world and need a grounding practice that strengthens both the body and mind while fostering clarity, focus, and resilience.
- You once practiced yoga but lost touch due to the overwhelming choices of activities available today and seek a consistent, meaningful, and effective approach to bringing yoga and meditation practice back in life now.
- You crave mental peace amidst the chaos of daily life, whether as a corporate leader, entrepreneur, or full-time parent, and need a practice that nurtures both mental serenity and physical vitality.

Who am I and why did I write this book?

My name is Vaibhavi Haridas and I was born Vaibhavi Agwan in Thane, Maharashtra. By profession, I am a Mechanical Engineer with two Master's degrees—in Technology and Business Administration—and a career spanning 18+ years as a technology leader in Corporate America. The United States is my adopted motherland, but my heart and soul remain deeply rooted in India—the land that nurtured my spiritual foundation.

My journey: From Childhood Practice to Lifelong Devotion

My connection to yoga and meditation began early in childhood. At Holy Cross Convent High School, our Principal, Sister Rosita, introduced us to daily meditation sessions broadcast over the PA (Public Announcement) system, embedding a deep sense of stillness and intrigue in me. During our physical training classes, I had the privilege of learning yoga from Nikam Sir, an exceptional teacher who instilled discipline and reverence for the practice.

Outside of school, I trained in *Rope Mallakhamb*, a traditional Indian sport that involves performing yoga postures while suspended on a rope- 20-foot in air. This developed my strength, flexibility, and love for asanas. As a gymnast, I relished the challenge of perfecting backflips and cartwheels, but like many students in the late '90s in India, the environment around me automatically put a pause on my passions to focus on academic excellence and board exams.

Fast forward 15 years, two kids, and a demanding corporate career later—I found myself drawn back to the roots of my practice. Although I had always maintained a daily *Surya Namaskar* routine, I felt an undeniable pull to deepen my understanding. This led me to immerse myself in the ancient Hindu philosophy. I took a Foundations of *Vedanta* course offered by Chinmaya Mission to formalize my understanding and also started studying the philosophy of the *Bhagwat Geeta*- this became a guiding force in my life.

A few years later, another turning point came when my sister, Aniketa, introduced me to the concept of Yoga Teacher Training Certification. This was the missing piece—I realized that my passion for yoga was not just personal but something I wanted to share with others. And then right during peak of COVID, there was a divine intervention that led me to take a leap and establish a non-profit organization called Arva Yoga. You can read about Arva Yoga and the divine intervention story in a section dedicated to it at the end of the book.

Balancing Yoga with Corporate Leadership

For the past two decades, I have held leadership roles across various industries, starting my career in USA as a Business Analyst in 2005 and then progressing through various roles of progressive responsibility from Project Manager, Product Manager, Business Transformation Lead, Director, Vice President, and finally, Senior Vice President. In my most recent role, I led a team of 180 technologists—

managing complex projects, high-pressure decision-making, and the relentless pace of corporate life.

I know firsthand the challenges of high-performance environments, where stress, deadlines, and expectations can feel overwhelming. Through all of this, my yoga practice became my anchor. I learned that success in the corporate world isn't just about hard skills and strategies—it requires mental clarity, emotional resilience, and a sense of inner peace.

Taking another leap

As a technology leader, my career has always been fast-paced and demanding. But in 2024, I chose to step back and embrace something I hadn't prioritized in years: time. Time with my family, time to reflect, and time to create. What began as a sabbatical to simply be present with my kids turned into a year of profound joy, creativity, and growth—for all of us.

The year started with a deeply personal project: launching a small handicrafts business in memory of my grandmother: Ethnik Edge. It was my way of honoring her legacy while channeling my creativity. My teenagers joined me wholeheartedly, brainstorming prototypes and experimenting with designs. What began as a family bonding activity evolved into a crash course in entrepreneurship for them—and a chance for me to teach life skills that can't be learned in classrooms.

This entrepreneurial journey sparked another idea: a mini-MBA program for high school students during summer break. Leveraging my LinkedIn network, I was fortunate to recruit eight executives, each with MBAs from top U.S. business schools, to lead sessions based on a curriculum I drafted. The program was a hit. It culminated in a children's business fair, where 20 kids launched 12 businesses—several of which turned profitable within months. Watching their transformation and burgeoning confidence was nothing short of inspiring.

For my own business, the highlight of the year was a red-carpet moment: our product was featured in the Emmy's gift basket. Winning an innovation award was the cherry on top. What began as a tribute to my grandmother blossomed into a platform for creativity, recognition, and growth beyond anything I had envisioned.

Beyond business, 2024 was also about community. My nonprofit work flourished, starting with the Saree Run, where this year alone we raised over $15,000 for women's causes. Partnering with another nonprofit to organize our first yoga festival was a dream come true. Despite the 95-degree heat, 150+ attendees participated, including the General Counsel of India, adding a special touch to the event. Local studios led sessions, and my kids, along with their friends, pitched in behind the scenes, making it a true community effort.

An unexpected highlight was leading a fundraiser for my daughter's volleyball team. Having spent years writing checks for causes without fully understanding the effort behind them, this experience deepened my appreciation for grassroots community work. Together, we raised over $20,000 for various social causes in 2024, with exciting collaborations already in the works for 2025.

The most profound reward, however, has been the simple act of being present—reading a college essay, discussing dreams, or just listening to my kids speak their minds. These quiet moments reminded me of the beauty of slowing down.

This year reaffirmed the transformative power of stepping back to reconnect, reflect, and create. I also was encouraged this year to start regular yoga classes and from this yet another venture was born- Ethnik Yoga!

Looking ahead

I hope this glimpse into my journey gives you a deeper understanding of who I am and why I feel an unwavering call to share this knowledge with the world. When you've walked a path—felt its struggles, its breakthroughs, its transformation—you don't just keep it to yourself. As an empath, I feel a profound responsibility to light the way for others, making their journey smoother, their growth faster, and their transformation even more powerful. Because knowledge isn't meant to be kept—it's meant to be shared, so we can all rise together. Today, through Arva Yoga and Ethnik Yoga platforms, I share this SHIVA technique and power of 5-4-3-2-1 methodology of yoga and meditation with the world, leading daily and weekly online sessions that seamlessly weave ancient practices into modern living.

This book is the culmination of that journey—a method that has deeply transformed my life and one that I know holds the power to transform yours. And it's 108 pages by design- The number symbolizing the cosmic journey to the divine: 1 representing the Supreme Consciousness or SHIVA, 0 signifying unity and infinity, and 8 embodying the five elements along with mind, intellect, and ego. Together, they reflect the connection between the individual and the universe, integrating the physical, mental, and spiritual realms. **Om Namah Shivaya.**

FOREWARD

I feel happy and honored to write the foreword for this exceptional yoga book, " SHIVA - The 5 sacred steps to success and serenity" authored by Vaibhavi Haridas. Apart from a successful professional and a compassionate mother she is dedicated to help the humanity through teaching yoga and other creative arts.

As a practitioner and teacher of Kriya yoga for 31 years, I have experienced firsthand the transformative power of this ancient yoga practice. Yoga as often misunderstood as some physical exercise is actually integration of body, mind and spirit which leads to healthy body, serene mind and sharp intellect. In this book, Vaibhavi delves deep into the philosophy and practice of yoga, offering readers a comprehensive guide to achieving physical, mental, and spiritual well-being. The most interesting part of this book is a unique blending of ancient yogic practice with the attributes of Lord Shiva who has taught Yoga, Tantra, and Grammar in the ancient time. The methodical and simple techniques of 5-4-3-2-1 method yoga in this book would be a practical guide for not only the professionals but also people from all walks of society to be free from stress, give strength to overcome physical and mental challenges and achieve a successful goal-oriented life. The journey that led to the creation of this book is a testament to Vaibhavi's dedication and passion for yoga.

Personally, yoga has been a source of immense peace and all-round growth in my life. It has helped me cultivate calmness, resilience, and a deeper connection to Divine and the world around me. I am confident that readers will find similar benefits as they explore the pages of this book.

Vaibhavi has poured her heart and soul into this work, and it shines through every chapter which will take the readers to a new understanding of Lord Shiva and Yoga. The clarity, depth, and wisdom contained within these pages make it a must-read for anyone seeking to enrich their lives through yoga.

I encourage you to embrace the teachings of this book and embark on your own journey of self- discovery and transformation. Let this book be your guide as you explore the profound practice of yoga and its benefits.

May the blessings of Lord Shiva the supreme yogi be upon all of us,

Swami Atmavidyananda Giri

Kriya Yoga Institute, USA

February 2025

TABLE OF CONTENTS

Part 1:

The SHIVA Technique

(Philosophical Foundation)

Shloka:

शिवाय नमः परमकारणकारणाय ।

दिव्याय देवाय दिगम्बराय ।।

(Shivāya namaḥ paramakāraṇakāraṇāya,

divyāya devāya digambarāya.)

Translation:

"Salutations to Shiva, the ultimate cause of all causes,

The divine, the formless, the eternal."

Source: Shiva Mahimna Stotra

Shiva—the cosmic dancer, the silent meditator, the fierce warrior, and the compassionate father—is a paradox in motion, embodying both the stillness of the Himalayas and the dynamic energy of the cosmos. His essence is not confined to myths and temples; it is a blueprint for modern life, offering wisdom that applies to every role we play—whether as professionals, leaders, spouses, parents, or seekers of truth.

In today's fast-paced, high-pressure world, many corporate workers and executives struggle to balance ambition with inner peace, decision-making with ethics, and success with humility. Many parents and spouses grapple with navigating responsibilities while staying present and connected. Shiva, in his multifaceted existence, provides a timeless ideal—one that seamlessly integrates into modern life and corporate culture.

This section explores the philosophical depth of Shiva's attributes and how embracing them can transform us into effective leaders, mindful partners and parents, and fulfilled individuals.

Introduction of SHIVA

Shiva: The Perfect Corporate Leader

In the competitive world of business, success often comes at the cost of mental peace, integrity, and work-life balance. Shiva, however, teaches us that true leadership is about balance, foresight, and resilience.

1. The Visionary (Third Eye of Perception)

A great leader, like Shiva, must see beyond the immediate—the ability to anticipate trends, make long-term decisions, and remain focused despite distractions.

Shiva's third eye symbolizes clarity and perception—a trait crucial for any executive who must sift through chaos and see the bigger picture.

2. Mastery Over Ego (Vairagya – Detachment Without Apathy)

Shiva is known for his vairagya (detachment)—he remains unaffected by praise or blame, success or failure.

A corporate leader who can detach from personal biases, ego-driven decisions, and office politics is far more effective in managing teams and making rational, strategic decisions.

This balance is essential for workplace harmony, conflict resolution, and innovation.

3. Balance Between Dynamism & Stillness (Tandava & Meditation)

Shiva embodies both tandava (dynamic action) and meditation (deep reflection).

The best executives understand that action must be followed by introspection—rushed decisions without reflection lead to burnout, while excessive contemplation without execution results in stagnation.

4. Emotional Intelligence & Equanimity (Neelkanth – The Poison Swallower)

In the legend of Samudra Manthan, Shiva drank the halahala (poison) to save the world but held it in his throat (thereby gaining the name of Neelkanth- the one with blue throat), neither letting it harm him nor others.

In corporate life, a great leader absorbs workplace toxicity (stress, pressure, conflicts) without letting it affect their decision-making or their teams negatively.

5. Leading with Ethics & Integrity (Dharmic Leadership)

In today's corporate world, ethical leadership is often sacrificed for short-term gains. Shiva represents dharma (righteousness) and fearlessness—qualities of leaders who stand by their principles, inspire loyalty, and cultivate trust.

Shiva: The Ideal Husband & Partner

Shiva's relationship with Parvati is a profound example of respect, balance, and divine love—qualities that make him an ideal husband and life partner.

1. Equal Partnership & Mutual Growth

Unlike many deities, Shiva does not place himself above Parvati. He treats her as an equal—both spiritually and intellectually.

In an ideal relationship, growth is mutual—both partners empower, challenge, and evolve together rather than one dominating the other.

2. Respect for Independence

Shiva never imposes his will upon Parvati. In a modern relationship, allowing space for individual growth while nurturing a partnership is key.

A true partner does not control but rather inspires their spouse to reach their highest potential.

3. Emotional Depth & Devotion

Shiva's devotion to Parvati is unwavering—he is deeply involved yet unattached, passionate yet centered.

In any successful relationship, one must be fully present yet not possessive, deeply connected yet respectful of individuality.

4. Overcoming Differences with Wisdom

Parvati's love is filled with moments of disagreement, but Shiva responds with patience and wisdom.

Every relationship has conflicts—but true love is not about eliminating them; it is about transcending them through understanding and growth.

Shiva: The Perfect Father & Guide

Shiva is not just a cosmic force—he is also a nurturing father to Ganesha and Kartikeya, embodying the ideal qualities of parenthood and mentorship.

1. Allowing Freedom & Learning Through Experience

Shiva does not force his beliefs on his children; instead, he allows them to discover their own paths.

The best parents are not those who control their children but those who empower them to think, explore, and develop their unique strengths.

2. Teaching by Example, Not Just Words

Shiva lives his values—whether it is discipline, compassion, or wisdom—and leads by example.

Children learn best not from instructions but from observing how their parents navigate challenges with grace.

3. Unconditional Love & Acceptance

Shiva never abandons or rejects his children, even when they make mistakes.

The greatest gift a parent can give is unconditional love—providing guidance without judgment, discipline without harshness, and presence without suffocation.

4. Encouraging Strength & Resilience

Shiva trains Kartikeya to be a warrior and prepares Ganesha for wisdom.

Great parenting involves recognizing each child's strengths and fostering an environment where they can thrive—whether in academics, creativity, leadership, or self-exploration.

Shiva: The Blueprint for a Perfect Human Being

Beyond corporate leadership, marriage, and parenting, Shiva stands as the ideal for human perfection based on these aspects of life and much more.

1. Balance Between Material & Spiritual Life

Shiva is both a yogi and a householder—he teaches that one does not need to renounce the world to attain enlightenment.

A balanced life includes both external success (career, family, relationships) and inner fulfillment (self-awareness, meditation, personal growth).

2. Mastery Over Desires (Not Repression, But Transcendence)

Shiva enjoys the world—he loves, dances, and engages—but is not bound by desires.

The ideal human is one who lives fully but is not enslaved by attachments or materialistic pursuits.

3. Compassion & Strength in Harmony

Shiva is both the destroyer and the protector, fierce yet deeply compassionate.

The truly evolved person is one who can be strong without arrogance, kind without weakness, and wise without condescension.

4. Embracing Imperfection & Growth

Shiva is known as Bholenath—the innocent one—because he does not hold onto grudges, anger, or ego.

True perfection is not about never making mistakes, but about evolving, forgiving, and growing beyond limitations.

Shiva is not just an ancient deity—he is a living ideal for anyone seeking a meaningful, successful, and balanced life. Whether in corporate leadership, relationships, parenthood, or self-mastery, the wisdom of Shiva provides a roadmap for harmonizing ambition with peace, power with humility, and action with wisdom.

By understanding and embodying Shiva's principles, we can transform not only ourselves but also the world around us.

Step onto the path.

Chapter 1

Sacred Steps to Transformation

Introduction to the SHIVA Framework and Its Connection to Ancient Wisdom

Shloka:
"योगश्चित्तवृत्तिनिरोधः" (Yogaś citta-vṛtti-nirodhaḥ)
Meaning:
"Yoga is the stilling of the fluctuations of the mind."

Source: Patanjali Yoga Sutras (1.2)

This verse from the Yoga Sutras of Patanjali sets the foundation for the SHIVA framework. Transformation begins with inner stillness, a quieting of mental turbulence, which allows one to harness energy, set clear intentions, and align with a higher purpose. The SHIVA technique simplifies these steps in a structured way, bridging ancient yogic wisdom with modern needs.

SHIVA: The 5 Pillars of Transformation

Transformation is at the heart of the yogic path, and few deities embody this concept more powerfully than Lord Shiva. He is the cosmic force of destruction and renewal, the stillness in meditation, and the fire of inner awakening. The SHIVA framework is a modern, structured approach inspired by this ancient wisdom—a five-step method designed to help professionals and seekers alike achieve balance, success, and serenity in their lives.

This is the framework for transformation through movement, breath, sound, stillness, and awareness, while reflecting Shiva's divine symbolism in yogic practice. SHIVA is an acronym that represents the five fundamental pillars of transformation:

S – Shavasana & Stillness – The three minutes of deep restoration that integrate the benefits of yoga, calm the nervous system, and allow true surrender—mirroring Shiva's meditative state.

H – Hatha & Harmony – The five sacred asanas that balance strength and flexibility, reflecting the union of Shiva's dual aspects—stillness & dynamism.

I – Inner Fire & Invocation – The four rounds of Surya Namaskar that awaken Tapas (discipline & transformation), much like Shiva's cosmic dance of creation and dissolution.

V – Vibration & Voice – The two chants or mantras that purify the mind and elevate consciousness, resonating with Shiva's Damaru (cosmic drum) and sacred sound 'Om'.

A – Awareness & Alignment – The single powerful intention (Sankalpa) that aligns thoughts, actions, and goals—mirroring Shiva's unwavering focus as the Adiyogi (first yogi).

Each of these elements corresponds to a core principle of yoga and self-realization, drawing upon ancient practices to create a simple, structured methodology that fits seamlessly into modern life.

The Link to Lord Shiva and Yogic Tradition

Lord Shiva is revered as Adi Yogi, the first yogi, who imparted the wisdom of yoga to the Saptarishis (Seven Sages). His form represents the perfect union of opposites—stillness and movement, destruction and renewal, meditation and action. The SHIVA framework is inspired by these dualities, helping practitioners integrate stillness with purpose-driven action in their daily lives.

In Hindu tradition, the number five holds deep significance, aligning with the Pancha Bhootas(Five Elements: Earth, Water, Fire, Air, and Space), which govern the body and mind. Shiva himself is often depicted with five heads, representing his omniscience and mastery over these forces. The 5-4-3-2-1 Method within this framework builds upon this sacred numerical foundation, offering a practical way to harmonize the body, breath, and mind.

A Bridge Between Ancient Wisdom and Modern Success

For centuries, yogis have sought spiritual liberation through these timeless practices. Today, professionals face a different kind of challenge—overwhelming stress, mental fatigue, and a constant struggle to find work-life balance. The SHIVA framework brings the wisdom of the ancients into the modern world, offering a structured yet flexible approach to transformation.

Through simple but profound daily rituals, practitioners can unlock clarity, cultivate resilience, and realign with their true purpose. Whether you are a seasoned yogi or a working professional looking for an effective way to integrate wellness into your routine, the SHIVA framework is your guide to achieving both external success and inner peace. Transformation begins with a single step. May this journey bring you closer to balance, wisdom, and the infinite energy of Shiva within.

Transformation starts within.

Chapter 2

The Power of Five – Understanding the Sacred Structure of the SHIVA Framework

Shloka:
पञ्चमहाभूतसंयुक्तं शरीरं योगिनां तपः ।
(Pañca-mahābhūta-saṁyuktaṁ śarīraṁ yogināṁ tapaḥ.)

Translation:
"The body, composed of the five great elements,
Becomes purified through yogic discipline."

Source: Shiva Purana

The SHIVA framework's 5 elements (asanas, breath, mantra, stillness, and intention) reflect the five forces of existence—Earth, Water, Fire, Air, and Space.

The Power of Five

In Hindu philosophy, five is not just a number—it is a cosmic blueprint. The Panchatattva (five elements) make up our physical being, the Panchakoshas (five sheaths) represent our subtle layers of existence, and even Lord Shiva himself manifests in five powerful aspects: Sadyojāta (Creation), Vāmadeva (Preservation), Aghora (Dissolution), Tatpurusha (Concealment), and Īshāna (Revelation).

This inherent structure of five mirrors the SHIVA technique, where each practice is designed to harmonize different aspects of life.

- **Five Asanas** – Representing strength, flexibility, and alignment of the body.
- **Four Sun Salutations** – Symbolizing breath-linked movement and life force activation.
- **Three Minutes of Shavasana** – The gateway to deep relaxation and surrender.
- **Two Chants** – Harnessing vibrational energy to cultivate focus and serenity.
- **One Intention** – A single-pointed focus to direct the mind and actions.

By practicing this 5-4-3-2-1 approach, we are, in essence, aligning ourselves with the cosmic rhythms, balancing the Panchatattva within, and invoking the wisdom of Lord Shiva—the ultimate embodiment of equilibrium and transcendence.

This method is not just a sequence of movements; it is a sacred process of transformation. Just as Shiva dances the Tandava, creating and dissolving worlds, we too undergo a daily cycle of renewal through this structured practice.

Bridging Science and Spirituality

Interestingly, modern neuroscience aligns with this ancient five-step approach. Studies on habit formation and neuroplasticity reveal that structured, repetitive practice builds new neural pathways, allowing individuals to form sustainable habits. The 5-4-3-2-1 method works in harmony with the brain's ability to adapt, focus, and thrive.

By grounding our practice in five interconnected steps, we create a repeatable, efficient, and transformative method that fosters both spiritual elevation and practical success.

As you move forward, reflect on this sacred structure. The universe itself functions in harmonious cycles—so why shouldn't we?

Balance is the key.

Chapter 3

Awakening Energy – The Role of Breath and Movement in Transformation

Shloka:

"प्राणायामेन युक्तेन सर्वरोगक्षयो भवेत्।"

(Prāṇāyāmena yuktena sarvarogakṣayo bhavet.)

Meaning:

"With controlled breath (pranayama), all diseases are destroyed."

Source: Hatha Yoga Pradipika (2.16)

Breath is life. The ancient yogic scriptures repeatedly emphasize the power of prana (life force energy) in shaping our well-being. Breath control through pranayama and coordinated movement through asanas and Surya Namaskars (Sun Salutations) are vital tools for aligning body, mind, and spirit. In the SHIVA technique, breath and movement serve as the bridge between the physical and the metaphysical, allowing us to harness energy for transformation.

Breath: The Unseen Power of Life

Every inhale we take draws in energy; every exhale releases stagnation. Yet, most of us breathe unconsciously, missing out on the profound effects of mindful respiration. The yogis discovered centuries ago that conscious breathing controls the mind, stabilizes emotions, and enhances mental clarity.

Scientific research supports this. Studies have shown that slow, deep breathing activates the parasympathetic nervous system, reducing stress hormones and fostering relaxation. Conversely, erratic, shallow breaths trigger the fight-or-flight response, leading to anxiety and fatigue.

The SHIVA framework integrates this wisdom through Surya Namaskars and Shavasana, ensuring that movement is always guided by breath, leading to:

- Improved focus and energy levels
- Reduced stress and anxiety
- Greater resilience in high-pressure situations

Movement: Aligning the Physical and Subtle Bodies

In yoga, movement is never random—it follows the rhythm of the breath. Surya Namaskar (Sun Salutation) is a perfect example of how movement, when synchronized with breath, becomes a sacred dance of energy.

Performing four rounds of Surya Namaskars in the SHIVA method is intentional. The number four represents stability, just as four directions hold the world in balance.

Through these salutations, we:

- Stretch and strengthen the body
- Improve circulation and detoxification
- Cultivate a moving meditation

Each posture in Surya Namaskar corresponds to an aspect of the Panchatattva (five elements):

1. Earth (Prithvi) – Grounding postures like mountain pose (Tadasana).
2. Water (Jala) – Flowing transitions between poses.
3. Fire (Agni) – Heat-generating postures like upward-facing dog.
4. Air (Vayu) – The breathwork involved in transitions.
5. Space (Akasha) – The expansion and openness we create in the body.

By practicing mindful movement and breathwork, we awaken dormant energy, improve vitality, and build resilience—all essential for success in both personal and professional life.

A Practical Application: Breath Awareness for Success

For busy professionals, stress often leads to mental fatigue, poor decision-making, and lack of clarity. Here's a simple breath-awareness practice you can do anytime:

- Pause whatever you are doing.
- Close your eyes and take a slow, deep breath in through your nose.
- Exhale fully through your mouth, letting go of tension.
- Repeat for five breaths, focusing only on the air moving in and out.

This micro-practice alone can reset your nervous system, bring you back to the present moment, and give you the clarity needed to handle challenges with ease.

Harnessing the Power of Prana

Breath and movement are not just physical activities—they are powerful tools for transformation. By understanding how they work together, we gain control over our energy, emotions, and thoughts.

As you move through the SHIVA technique, let each breath be intentional. Let each movement be purposeful. The mind, body, and spirit are always in dynamic conversation—and by listening to this dialogue, you align yourself with the greater rhythm of the universe.

Breathe. Flow. Expand.

Chapter 4

Inner Silence – The Power of Meditation and Stillness

Shloka:

योगश्चित्तवृत्तिनिरोधः ।।

(Yogaś citta-vṛtti-nirodhaḥ.)

Translation:

"Yoga is the cessation of the fluctuations of the mind."

Source: Patanjali's Yoga Sutras (1.2)

Inner silence is a key element of the SHIVA framework, where stillness leads to clarity and transformation. Ancient yogis discovered that when we cultivate inner stillness, we access a deeper intelligence beyond logic and emotions. This is where true creativity, clarity, and decision-making power reside.

The Noise of the World vs. The Silence Within

We live in an era of constant distractions—emails, notifications, deadlines, social media. The mind is like a monkey, constantly jumping from one thought to another. But wisdom arises in silence.

Modern neuroscience confirms this—meditation rewires the brain, strengthening areas responsible for focus, emotional regulation, and problem-solving while reducing stress-related brain activity.

Yet, most professionals struggle to meditate because they believe they "don't have time" or that their mind "won't stop thinking." The truth? Meditation is not about stopping thoughts—it is about observing them without attachment.

The SHIVA Approach to Meditation: Practical and Powerful

In the SHIVA framework, meditation is simple yet effective. A structured approach ensures maximum benefits in minimal time, making it ideal for busy professionals.

The practice includes:

Three Minutes of Shavasana (Corpse Pose) – A state of deep relaxation that prepares the mind for stillness.

Two Chants – Vibrational sound practices to center the mind and elevate consciousness.

One Clear Intention – A daily mental focus to align thoughts and actions.

By following this sequence, even five minutes of daily practice can shift your entire state of mind.

The Science of Stillness: Why It Works

- Meditation Lowers Stress – Studies show that regular meditation reduces cortisol (the stress hormone) and enhances resilience in high-pressure situations.
- Boosts Focus & Productivity – Professionals who meditate report greater concentration, faster decision-making, and reduced mental fatigue.
- Enhances Emotional Intelligence – By increasing self-awareness, meditation helps you navigate office politics, interpersonal conflicts, and leadership challenges with clarity and composure.
- Strengthens the Nervous System – Meditation activates the parasympathetic nervous system, promoting deep rest and rejuvenation.

A Simple Meditation for Instant Clarity

Try this one-minute meditation whenever you feel overwhelmed:

- Close your eyes and take a deep breath in.
- Exhale slowly, releasing any tension.
- Mentally repeat: "I am calm. I am centered. I am in control."
- Stay in stillness for a few breaths, then open your eyes.

Even this brief practice can reset your mind, bringing clarity and focus.

Stillness: The Secret to Lasting Success

Meditation is not just for monks in the Himalayas. It is for leaders, professionals, and anyone seeking balance in a chaotic world.

In the SHIVA technique, meditation is a non-negotiable practice—a way to align with the universe's rhythm, calm the mind, and make better decisions with effortless ease. Embrace stillness. In that silence, you will hear the whispers of your highest self-guiding you toward success and serenity.

Silence speaks wisdom.

Chapter 5

Vibrational Energy – The Power of Sound and Mantras

Shloka:
ओंकारं बिंदुसंयुक्तं नित्यं ध्यायंति योगिनः ।
(Oṁkāraṁ bindu-saṁyuktaṁ nityaṁ dhyāyanti yoginaḥ.)

Translation:
"Yogis continuously meditate on Om,
The cosmic sound united with divine consciousness."

Source: Mandukya Upanishad

Sound vibrations like OM cleanse the mind and align energy with the higher self, reinforcing SHIVA's mantra practice. Sound is not just a form of communication—it is energy in motion. In yogic tradition, mantras and chants have been used for centuries to elevate consciousness, enhance focus, and dissolve negative patterns. Modern science confirms that sound vibrations influence brainwaves, affecting mood, cognition, and even physical health. In the SHIVA technique, vibrational energy is harnessed through two chants that help align the mind, body, and spirit.

The Universe is Made of Sound

Ancient Hindu philosophy describes Nada Brahma—the belief that the universe itself is sound (nada), and sound is divine (Brahma). The primordial vibration Om (AUM) is said to be the source of all creation. Science echoes this idea: everything in existence vibrates at a frequency, including our thoughts and emotions.

When we chant, we are not merely producing sound—we are tuning our body and mind to higher frequencies, much like adjusting a musical instrument.

Mantras: The Science of Sacred Sounds

The word "mantra" comes from "man" (mind) and "tra" (tool or vehicle)—literally, a tool to train the mind. Mantras work by:

- Rewiring Neural Pathways – Repeating a mantra creates new, positive mental patterns, much like affirmations.
- Calming the Nervous System – Sound vibrations slow brainwave activity, inducing a meditative state.
- Boosting Focus & Resilience – Chanting stabilizes emotions, enhances clarity, and promotes self-confidence.
- Raising Energy Levels – High-frequency sounds uplift mood, reduce fatigue, and increase inner strength.

The SHIVA method integrates two simple yet powerful chants into daily practice, allowing busy professionals to tap into vibrational energy effortlessly.

The SHIVA Approach: Two Simple Chants for Daily Balance

Incorporating mantra chanting does not require hours of practice. Just two short chants daily can bring profound transformation.

Chant 1: Om Namah Shivaya (ॐ नमः शिवाय)

One of the most powerful Vedic mantras, it translates to "I bow to Shiva"—a call to inner wisdom and transformation.

Benefits: Calms the mind, enhances self-awareness, dissolves ego, and aligns with higher consciousness.

Chant 2: Gayatri Mantra (गायत्री मंत्र)

"ॐ भूर्भुवः स्वः ।

तत्सवितुर्वरेण्यं ।

भर्गो देवस्य धीमहि ।

धियो यो नः प्रचोदयात् ।।"

Meaning: "We meditate upon the divine light of the Supreme Being, may it illuminate our intellect."

Benefits: Boosts mental clarity, enhances decision-making, and strengthens intuition.

Even five minutes of chanting daily can help professionals sharpen focus, increase resilience, and maintain emotional balance in high-pressure environments. These are just two options but you can simply chant "Om" out loud for the same benefits.

The Power of Your Own Voice

Chanting isn't just about reciting words—it is about feeling the vibration resonate within. Your voice is your own healing instrument.

Try this simple sound meditation:

- Close your eyes and take a deep breath.
- As you exhale, softly chant "Om" and feel the vibration in your chest.
- Repeat for five rounds, allowing the sound to dissolve stress and bring clarity.
- This micro-practice is a game-changer—a quick way to reset your mind and re-align with your goals.

Unlocking Success with Sound

Most professionals underestimate the power of sound in shaping reality. But leaders, entrepreneurs, and visionaries across history have relied on affirmations, prayers, and chants to manifest success and clarity.

Incorporating two daily chants into the SHIVA technique is a simple yet profound way to access the ancient wisdom of vibration, helping you unlock mental peace, focus, and personal power—all in a matter of minutes.

Begin today. Chant. Vibrate. Transform.

Resonate with the universe.

Chapter 6

Inner Stillness – The Art of Mindful Silence

Shloka:
नैषा तर्केण मतिरापनेया ।
(Naiṣā tarkeṇa matirāpaneyā.)

Translation:
"This realization is not attained by mere logic,
But by direct inner experience."

Source: Katha Upanishad (1.2.23)

Stillness leads to deeper intuition and wisdom, beyond intellectual reasoning. In the midst of life's noise—career demands, family responsibilities, and social obligations—silence is the forgotten key to self-mastery. Modern professionals often seek external validation, but true clarity and success come from inner stillness. The SHIVA technique emphasizes the power of mindful silence as a means to sharpen focus, enhance resilience, and achieve mental peace.

Why Silence is Power

In Hindu philosophy, silence (mauna) is not just the absence of speech—it is a state of heightened awareness. The great sages, from Adi Shankaracharya to Swami Vivekananda, have emphasized that wisdom emerges not from constant thought, but from the stillness between thoughts.

Even neuroscience agrees—practicing silence for even a few minutes daily leads to:

- Stronger decision-making abilities – A quiet mind processes information more effectively.
- Better emotional regulation – Silence lowers stress hormone levels, reducing anxiety.
- Enhanced creativity – The brain makes deeper connections when it is not overstimulated.

Silence is not passive—it is active engagement with your inner world.

The SHIVA Approach: The 3-Minute Stillness Practice

The 5-4-3-2-1 Method integrates three minutes of silence daily as an essential reset for the nervous system. It is a simple yet powerful ritual that anyone—especially high achievers—can incorporate.

How to Practice Inner Stillness in 3 Minutes:

- Find a Quiet Space – This can be in your office, home, or even a park.
- Close Your Eyes – Shut out external distractions.
- Breathe Deeply – Inhale for four counts, exhale for four counts.
- Observe Without Reacting – Notice thoughts as they arise but do not engage.
- Return to the Present – When your mind drifts, gently bring it back to the breath.

This simple micro-practice rewires the brain for calm, clarity, and control, making it one of the most effective tools for success-oriented individuals.

The Science Behind Stillness

Modern research confirms what yogic wisdom has long taught: moments of silence allow the brain's default mode network (DMN) to activate, which is responsible for:

- Deep problem-solving
- Self-reflection and goal-setting
- Long-term memory consolidation

Successful people—from Steve Jobs to Mahatma Gandhi—have all credited quiet reflection as their secret weapon.

Silence and the Divine Connection

Lord Shiva, the Adi Yogi (first yogi), is often depicted in deep meditation—eyes closed, mind absorbed in absolute stillness. His state represents pure consciousness (Chidakasha), a mind beyond noise, distraction, or conflict.

Practicing silence is a way to tap into that same energy, creating space for divine wisdom and self-realization to emerge.

Embrace the Power of Silence

In a world that glorifies constant activity, silence is your hidden superpower. Three minutes of stillness daily can help you make smarter decisions, stay emotionally resilient, and move through life with unwavering clarity.

Start today. Be still. Listen within. Transform.

Stillness is strength.

Chapter 7

Vision & Intention – Aligning with Your Higher Purpose

Shloka:

"संकल्पमात्रमेकं हि संसारस्य विमोचनम्।"

(Sankalpa-mātram ekaṁ hi saṁsārasya vimocanam.)

Meaning:

"A single, resolute intention is enough to liberate one from worldly bondage."

Source: Shiva Purana

True transformation begins with clarity of vision and intention. Every great leader, visionary, and spiritual seeker starts with a Sankalpa (a deep, conscious resolve). Lord Shiva, the supreme yogi, is known as the embodiment of focused intention—whether in meditation, cosmic dance, or the destruction of illusions. The SHIVA framework integrates this wisdom, guiding professionals and yogis alike to harness the power of focused intention to align their lives with their true purpose.

The Power of Vision & Sankalpa

In yogic and Vedic traditions, a Sankalpa is more than a goal—it is a soul-driven commitment to transformation. Unlike fleeting resolutions, a true Sankalpa is rooted in dharma (higher purpose) and acts as a bridge between thought and reality.

In modern terms, think of it as a powerful internal GPS:

- Directs your energy toward meaningful success
- Eliminates distractions and mental clutter
- Builds resilience and inner strength

Neuroscience backs this up—when you set a clear intention, the brain's reticular activating system (RAS) filters out distractions and focuses your mind on achieving the goal.

The SHIVA Technique: The 1-Intention Practice

The 5-4-3-2-1 Method integrates the power of intention as its final and most crucial step. Every session, every day, you commit to a single, focused intention. This primes your mind for success and helps you take aligned action.

How to Set Your Daily Intention in 1 Minute:

Pause & Breathe – Inhale deeply, exhale slowly.

Ask Yourself: "What is the most important thing I need today?"

Use Affirmations:

"I am focused and strong."

"I will bring clarity and confidence to my work."

"I act with purpose and balance."

Visualize Success – Picture yourself achieving your intention.

This simple ritual aligns your mind, body, and spirit toward purpose-driven success.

Ancient Wisdom Meets Modern Neuroscience

Studies show that intention-setting activates the prefrontal cortex, improving focus, emotional regulation, and decision-making. Successful entrepreneurs, athletes, and leaders use intention-setting as a secret tool for peak performance.

- Oprah Winfrey attributes her success to daily intention-setting.
- Steve Jobs used visualization and focused attention for Apple's innovation.
- Indian sages and yogis have long practiced Sankalpa for spiritual elevation.

The secret? They don't leave their success to chance—they create it with conscious intention.

Shiva: The Ultimate Master of Focused Intention

Lord Shiva's third eye is a symbol of supreme focus and insight. When open, it destroys ignorance; when closed, it sees the ultimate truth. This represents the power of single-pointed intention—when our vision is clear, nothing can stand in our way.

By incorporating daily intention-setting, we align ourselves with Shiva's wisdom—moving through life with purpose, clarity, and unwavering determination.

Step Into Your Power: Set Your Intention Today

Your energy flows where your intention goes. Whether in career, relationships, health, or personal growth, aligning with a higher purpose brings success effortlessly.

Take one minute today—pause, reflect, set your intention, and watch your world transform.

See it. Manifest it.

Chapter 8

Action & Detachment – The Dance of Effort and Surrender

Sacred Shloka:

"कर्मण्येवाधिकारस्ते मा फलेषु कदाचन। मा कर्मफलहेतुर्भूर्मा ते सङ्गोऽस्त्वकर्मणि॥"

Meaning:

"You have the right to perform your actions, but never to the fruits of your actions. Do not be attached to the results, nor remain inactive."

Source: Bhagavad Gita (2.47)

This shloka, one of the most profound teachings of Lord Krishna, aligns perfectly with Lord Shiva's philosophy. Shiva is both the ultimate ascetic, detached from worldly desires, and the cosmic dancer, fully engaged in creation and destruction. This balance between intense action and deep surrender is the foundation of the SHIVA technique.

Effort Without Attachment: The Secret to Success

In modern professional life, we often find ourselves trapped between over-effort and burnout, or passivity and inaction. The key to success lies in disciplined effort combined with non-attachment to outcomes. When we embrace action without obsession over results, we unlock true freedom and peak performance.

Modern psychology and neuroscience confirm that high performers, whether athletes, entrepreneurs, or spiritual seekers, excel when they detach from anxiety over results and focus on process-driven mastery.

- Surgeons perform best when they trust their skills instead of fearing failure.
- CEOs make confident decisions when they act from clarity rather than fear.
- Yogis reach deeper meditation states when they release expectations.

This is what Shiva embodies—total commitment to action while remaining completely free from ego-driven outcomes.

The SHIVA Approach: The Power of Focused Action

In the 5-4-3-2-1 Method, structured practice ensures that you:

- Show up daily with discipline
- Perform each step with full awareness
- Let go of attachment to immediate results

Rather than chasing perfection or fearing failure, you commit to the process, knowing results will follow naturally.

3-Step Action Framework:

1. Set Your Daily Goals with Clarity:

Choose one major task that aligns with your long-term vision.

Write it down with a firm yet flexible mindset.

2. Engage Fully Without Mental Resistance:

Avoid distractions and immerse yourself in the action.

Practice "flow state" by being present in the moment.

3. Detach & Trust the Process:

Remind yourself: "I act with full energy, but I release the outcome."

Accept that delays, failures, or deviations are all part of the journey.

This is the Shiva way of working—engage with your fullest potential, then let go, knowing that what is meant to be will unfold.

Shiva's Cosmic Dance: The Ultimate Balance of Action & Surrender

Lord Shiva's Tandava—the cosmic dance of creation and destruction—symbolizes the perfect interplay of effort and detachment. Every movement is powerful, yet he dances in absolute freedom, unattached to the outcome.

This is your key to success in life:

- Act with full energy, like Shiva in his dance.

- Let go of fear and over-analysis.
- Trust in the divine rhythm of life—everything unfolds at the right time.

By integrating this mindset, you will work smarter, not harder, avoid burnout, and experience greater fulfillment.

Surrender is Power, Not Weakness

Many professionals hesitate to let go because they equate surrender with passivity. But in truth, detachment gives you supreme power:

- Less stress – because you stop obsessing over outcomes.
- More confidence – because you trust yourself fully.
- Greater success – because you take bold action without fear of failure.

When you embrace both focused effort and fearless surrender, you become a true master of your destiny.

Daily Practice: Shiva's Law of Action & Detachment

Each day, before you start work or practice, affirm:

"I act with complete dedication and let go of attachment to results. I trust in the process and the divine flow of life."

This mindset shift will make you unstoppable.

By practicing the SHIVA framework, you are not just following a routine—you are awakening the divine wisdom and strength of Shiva within you. The 5-4-3-2-1 method is your modern Trishul, cutting through stress, confusion, and obstacles, leading to clarity and success.

Do, release, trust.

Part 2:

5-4-3-2-1 Methodology Explained

(SHIVA Technique in Action)

Shloka:
कायवाङ्गनसां यत्नः कारणं सिद्धये योगिनाम् ।।
(Kāya-vāṅ-manasāṁ yatnaḥ kāraṇaṁ siddhaye yogināṁ.)

Translation:
"The alignment of body, speech, and mind is the key to yogic mastery."

Source: Shiva Samhita

Shiva, the embodiment of transformation, balance, and transcendence, offers a practical pathway to self-mastery. The 5-4-3-2-1 Methodology, inspired by his divine wisdom, is a structured approach designed to integrate movement, breathwork, meditation, and intention-setting into daily life. More than just a sequence of practices, this framework serves as a spiritual and psychological reset—one that empowers busy professionals, dedicated yogis, and seekers alike to cultivate both inner peace and external success.

This system is not about adding another task to your already full schedule. Instead, it is a streamlined yet profoundly effective practice that aligns with your natural rhythms, helping you navigate the demands of modern life while staying deeply connected to yourself. By dedicating just a few minutes each day, this methodology enables you to unlock Shiva's essence within you—unshakable focus, resilience, and serenity.

This section explores how the philosophical elements discussed in the previous chapter can be put into action in form of 5-4-3-2-1 methodology to then transform us into effective leaders, mindful partner and parents,, and fulfilled individuals- all spending just 30 minutes a day!

Shiva as the Archetype of the 5-4-3-2-1 Methodology

The 5-4-3-2-1 practice mirrors Shiva's own cyclic process of creation, sustenance, transformation, dissolution, and renewal. Each step represents a crucial aspect of human evolution—physical, mental, energetic, and spiritual:

5 Sacred Movements – Strengthening the Body

Shiva's cosmic dance, Tandava, represents the rhythmic flow of the universe—a continuous cycle of creation and destruction. Just as movement is intrinsic to life, the first step in the methodology focuses on five essential categories of movement that realign the body:

- Standing Asanas – Grounding & Strength
- Seated Asanas – Stability & Reflection
- Quad/ On all fours Pose – Core Activation & Balance
- Supine/ On your back Asanas – Rejuvenation & Integration
- Prone/ on your belly Asanas – Deep Strength & Surrender

This practice removes stagnation, enhances energy circulation, and prepares the body for breathwork and meditation.

4 Sun Salutations – Awakening Inner Fire

The four rounds of Surya Namaskar (Sun Salutations) mirror the four cardinal directions and the cyclical nature of time—morning, noon, evening, and night. Shiva, the Aditya (Sun's energy) within us, fuels willpower, clarity, and transformation through this sequence. Practicing these rounds activates prana (life force), clears mental fog, and invigorates the entire system.

3 Minutes of Stillness – Shavasana for Integration

Shiva, as the great ascetic, demonstrates the power of absolute stillness (Samadhi). Without silence, movement is incomplete. Three minutes of deep stillness in Shavasana allow the body and mind to absorb the practice, integrating movement and breathwork into deep relaxation. This phase restores the nervous system and enhances focus and emotional balance.

2 Vibrational Chants – Harnessing the Power of Sound

The power of mantra and vibration is a core aspect of Shiva's presence. The chanting of 'Om' at the beginning and end of practice serves as a bridge between the gross (physical body) and the subtle (energy and mind). Other mantras, such as So Ham

(I am that) or universal affirmations, can be used for focus, mindfulness, and self-realization.

1 Powerful Intention – Aligning with Purpose

Shiva is the ultimate yogi, yet he also plays the role of a householder, protector, and cosmic guide. Setting an intention at the beginning of practice, whether for mental clarity, success, resilience, or emotional strength, anchors the entire sequence in personal meaning. Intentions are not passive thoughts but energetic blueprints that influence action.

Why This Practice Works: Science Meets Spirituality

The 5-4-3-2-1 Methodology is a fusion of ancient wisdom and modern neuroscience. It taps into the core principles of habit formation, neuroplasticity, and energy optimization, making it an ideal system for those seeking balance between external success and inner peace.

1. Activates the Parasympathetic Nervous System (Rest & Restore Mode)

- The combination of movement, breath, and stillness calms the nervous system, reducing stress hormones (cortisol) and enhancing focus.
- Just 15-20 minutes of mindful movement and breathwork can significantly improve productivity, emotional regulation, and overall well-being.

2. Enhances Neuroplasticity & Cognitive Function

- Asanas and breathwork enhance brain function, emotional resilience, and cognitive sharpness.
- Chanting and intention-setting strengthen neural pathways associated with discipline, focus, and self-confidence.

3. Aligns with the Body's Natural Energy Cycles

- The Sun Salutations invigorate the system, syncing bodily rhythms with circadian cycles.
- Shavasana and chanting ground energy and reset emotional patterns, leading to a more balanced, focused state.

4. Provides a Daily Reset for the Modern Professional

- Unlike long, complicated routines, this streamlined approach ensures that even busy professionals, parents, and leaders can maintain consistency.
- By incorporating movement, breath, stillness, sound, and intention, the mind-body system is recalibrated daily for optimal performance.

Shiva's Message: The Balance of Effort & Surrender

Shiva's dance (Tandava) is not just an act of destruction—it is a process of renewal and balance. This methodology reflects the same cosmic principles:

- Effort in Movement (Shakti) and Ease in Stillness (Shiva)
- Dynamism in Asanas and Serenity in Meditation
- Structure in Practice and Freedom in Intention

Incorporating the 5-4-3-2-1 methodology into daily life is a way of honoring both the divine and the practical within us. It is a system that prepares us for external challenges while strengthening inner resolve.

Awakening Your Inner Shiva

Shiva is not an external force—Shiva is you. Each time you step onto the mat, you engage in a sacred dialogue with your highest self. The 5-4-3-2-1 methodology is not merely a set of techniques; it is a living philosophy that can transform the way you move, think, breathe, and act.

By aligning movement, breath, stillness, sound, and intention, you create a harmonious daily ritual that supports clarity, purpose, and resilience.

In this practice, there is no perfection—only progress. There is no destination—only awakening.

Align body, align mind.

Chapter 9

The 5 Sacred Movements – The Role of Asanas in Body-Mind Alignment

Shloka:

शरीरमाद्यं खलु धर्मसाधनम् ।।

(Śarīram ādyaṁ khalu dharmasādhanam.)

Translation:

"The body is the first instrument for spiritual practice"

Source: Kumarasambhavam (Kālidāsa)

Physical movement (asanas) is not separate from spirituality—it is the foundation for higher awareness.

The Sacred Dance of Shiva: Moving into Alignment

Lord Shiva, the eternal yogi, embodies the perfect union of stillness and motion. His cosmic dance, the Tandava, represents the rhythm of the universe—the balance of destruction and creation, effort and surrender, movement and stillness. Just as Shiva moves in perfect harmony with the cosmos, we too must align our body, breath, and mind to experience true well-being.

In yoga, this alignment is achieved through the five sacred movements that correspond to the way energy flows within us:

1. Standing Asanas – Grounding & Strength
2. Seated Asanas – Stability & Reflection
3. All-Fours/Quad Pose – Core Activation & Balance
4. Supine Asanas – Rejuvenation & Integration
5. Prone Asanas – Deep Strength & Surrender

Each of these movements aligns with the 5-4-3-2-1 Methodology, ensuring a structured approach to physical, mental, and spiritual balance.

The 5 Sacred Movements: Asana Categories & Benefits

The following table organizes asanas into five major categories, covering a holistic range of spinal movements for complete body-mind integration. This is just a selection of asanas from the hundreds of asanas which I teach and practice in my daily classes but a good selection for a blend of novice and advanced yogis. If you are new to yoga, check the resources at the end of the book for additional resources.

Category	Asana Name (Sanskrit)	Asana Name (Indian/English)	Primary Benefits
Standing	Tadasana	Palm Tree Pose	Improves posture, balance, and awareness
Standing	Vrikshasana	Tree Pose	Enhances stability and concentration
Standing	Virabhadrasana I	Warrior I	Strengthens legs, core, and focus
Standing	Virabhadrasana II	Warrior II	Builds stamina and resilience
Standing	Utkatasana	Chair Pose	Engages thighs, boosts metabolism
Standing	Trikonasana	Triangle Pose	Opens hips, enhances lateral flexibility
Standing	Ardha Chandrasana	Half Moon Pose	Develops coordination and core strength
Standing	Parivrtta Trikonasana	Revolved Triangle Pose	Improves spinal flexibility, detoxifies organs
Standing	Padangusthasana	Big Toe Pose	Stretches hamstrings, soothes the nervous system
Standing	Garudasana	Eagle Pose	Enhances balance and mental clarity
Standing	Utkata Konasana	Goddess Pose	Strengthens legs, promotes feminine energy

Standing	Utthita Parsvakonasana	Extended Side Angle	Strengthens legs, opens hips
Seated	Padmasana	Lotus Pose	Prepares the mind for meditation
Seated	Sukhasana	Easy Pose	Encourages relaxation and groundedness
Seated	Paschimottanasana	Seated Forward Bend	Stretches spine, calms the mind
Seated	Baddha Konasana	Bound Angle Pose	Opens hips, improves digestion
Seated	Ardha Matsyendrasana	Half Spinal Twist	Enhances spinal flexibility, aids detoxification
All Fours (Quad Pose)	Marjariasana-Bitilasana	Cat-Cow	Improves spinal mobility, stimulates digestion
All Fours	Balasana	Child's Pose	Relieves stress, elongates the spine
All Fours	Vyaghrasana	Tiger Pose	Enhances Spinal Flexibility
All Fours	Chamatkarasana	Wild Thing	Builds strength in shoulders and upper back
All Fours	Parsva Balasana	Thread the Needle	Releases tension from shoulders and back
Supine	Savasana	Corpse Pose	Facilitates deep relaxation, integrates practice
Supine	Supta Baddha Konasana	Reclining Bound Angle	Enhances flexibility and circulation
Supine	Setu Bandhasana	Bridge Pose	Strengthens the spine, opens the chest

Supine	Viparita Karani	Legs-Up-The-Wall	Reduces stress, promotes lymphatic flow
Supine	Jathara Parivartanasana	Reclined Spinal Twist	Releases tension from the spine and shoulders
Prone	Bhujangasana	Cobra Pose	Strengthens the spine, expands the chest
Prone	Salabhasana	Locust Pose	Improves posture, builds lower back strength
Prone	Dhanurasana	Bow Pose	Enhances spinal flexibility, boosts energy
Prone	Makarasana	Crocodile Pose	Calms the nervous system, realigns the spine
Prone	Adho Mukha Svanasana	Downward-Facing Dog	Stretches the entire body, increases circulation

The 5 Directions of the Spine: A Balanced Approach

In yogic wisdom, spinal movement is key to energy flow (prana). To maintain spinal health and unlock higher consciousness, the five essential spinal movements must be practiced daily. Some examples of the five directions of the spine in asanas is below:

Spinal Direction	Asana Example	Primary Benefit
Extension (Inversion)	Adho Mukha Svanasana (Downward-Facing Dog)	Boosts circulation, improves posture
Forward Bend	Paschimottanasana (Seated Forward Bend)	Stretches spine, reduces anxiety
Backward Bend	Bhujangasana (Cobra Pose)	Strengthens back, opens heart chakra
Lateral Bend	Trikonasana (Triangle Pose)	Improves side flexibility, enhances balance

Twist	Ardha Matsyendrasana (Half Spinal Twist)	Detoxifies organs, improves spinal mobility

By integrating these five movements, we prevent energy blockages, release stiffness, and create a strong, supple spine—the pathway of Kundalini energy.

Applying the 5-4-3-2-1 Methodology

The 5-4-3-2-1 Method structures these sacred movements into a practical, accessible practice:

- 5 Sacred Movements (Standing, Seated, Quad, Supine, Prone)
- 4 Core Components (Breath, Alignment, Intention, Stillness)
- 3 Key Benefits (Physical Strength, Mental Clarity, Emotional Balance)
- 2 Anchors (Practice + Detachment)
- 1 Goal (Complete Integration of Body & Mind)

Sacred Flow: A Daily Practice Inspired by Shiva

Each day, before beginning your practice, invoke Lord Shiva by mentally chanting:

"ॐ नमः शिवाय।" (Om Namah Shivaya – I bow to the Divine within and beyond.)

Then, move through one asana from each category in five conscious breaths, focusing on stillness in motion—just like Shiva in his cosmic dance.

As you surrender into Savasana at the end of your practice, remember: Movement is prayer. Stillness is wisdom. Balance is liberation.

Through these five sacred movements, we align ourselves with the eternal rhythm of the universe and walk the path of transformation, strength, and peace—just as Shiva intended.

Move with purpose.

Chapter 10

The 4 Sun Salutations – Awakening Inner Fire Through Movement

The Sacred Practice of Surya Namaskar

Shloka:

सूर्याद्वै खल्विमानि भूतानि जायन्ते ।

(Sūryād vai khalv imāni bhūtāni jāyante.)

Translation:

"From the Sun, all beings are born."

Source: Chandogya Upanishad

Surya Namaskar honors the life-giving energy of the Sun and awakens inner radiance. The sun, known as Surya in Sanskrit, has been revered in Hindu philosophy as the ultimate source of energy, vitality, and consciousness. In yogic tradition, Surya Namaskar (Sun Salutation) is a dynamic sequence of asanas that honors this life-giving force, aligning the physical body with its pranic energy. Practicing Sun Salutations generates heat (Agni), stimulates circulation, and awakens prana (life force) within us, fostering strength, flexibility, and mental clarity.

The number four in the 5-4-3-2-1 methodology represents the four rounds of Sun Salutations practiced daily. This consistent rhythm of movement and breath synchronization ignites an internal transformation, preparing the body and mind for deeper meditative states. The repeated cycles of Sun Salutations help set a foundation for discipline, devotion, and a balanced nervous system, making them an integral part of this framework.

The 12-Step Hatha Surya Namaskar Sequence

Each round of Sun Salutations consists of 12 postures performed in a fluid motion, each linked with conscious inhalation and exhalation. Below is a breakdown of each step, including the Sanskrit names and their significance.

One Round of Surya Namaskar is a combination of 12 steps as described below:

Step	Pose Name (Sanskrit & English)	Description & Benefits
1	Pranamasana (Prayer Pose)	Stand tall with feet together, palms joined at the heart center. This pose cultivates grounding, gratitude, and intention-setting.
2	Hasta Uttanasana (Raised Arms Pose)	Inhale, lift arms overhead, arching slightly backward. This stretches the spine, engages the core, and opens the chest.
3	Uttanasana (Standing Forward Bend)	Exhale, fold forward, bringing hands toward the floor. Stretches hamstrings, stimulates digestion, and calms the mind.
4	Ashwa Sanchalanasana (Equestrian Pose)	Inhale, step the right leg back, lowering the knee. Opens the hips, strengthens legs, and enhances balance.
5	Dandasana/Phalakasana (Plank Pose)	Hold your breath for a moment, step the left leg back, keeping the body in a straight line. Builds core strength, stability, and endurance.
6	Ashtanga Namaskara (Eight-Limbed Salutation)	Exhale, Lower knees, chest, and chin to the ground. Strengthens arms, shoulders, and chest while grounding the body.
7	Bhujangasana (Cobra Pose)	Inhale, lift the chest, keeping elbows slightly bent. Opens the heart, strengthens the spine, and activates prana.
8	Adho Mukha Svanasana (Downward-Facing Dog)	Exhale, lift hips, creating an inverted "V" shape. Stretches the spine, hamstrings, and shoulders, promoting circulation.
9	Ashwa Sanchalanasana (Equestrian Pose)	Inhale, step the right foot forward, mirroring step 4. Improves flexibility and hip mobility.

10	Uttanasana (Standing Forward Bend)	Exhale, step the left foot forward, folding from the hips. Enhances blood flow to the brain and calms the nervous system.
11	Hasta Uttanasana (Raised Arms Pose)	Inhale, rise with arms lifted, arching slightly. Reawakens energy and expands lung capacity.
12	Pranamasana (Prayer Pose)	Exhale, return hands to heart center. Completes the cycle with gratitude and balance.

This 12-step process with right leg going back and coming forward completes one round of Surya Namaskar. Repeating the same exact 12 steps with now left leg going back in step 4 and bringing the left leg forward in step 9 will complete the second round. These two rounds together comprise a set of Surya Namaskar. Total of four rounds would equal to two sets of Surya Namaskar.

Why Four Rounds of Surya Namaskar Daily?

Performing four complete rounds of Sun Salutations daily allows for a well-rounded practice that balances body, mind, and spirit. Here's why this number holds significance for a 30 minute practice:

1. Physical Activation & Strength: Four rounds incorporate sufficient movement to warm up and strengthen the entire body without overexertion. This makes it an ideal practice for professionals with busy schedules.

2. Energy Flow & Chakra Alignment: The sequence engages all seven chakras, activating prana flow and ensuring a balanced energy system.

3. Mind-Body Synchronization: Breath awareness in each movement fosters mindfulness, reducing stress and enhancing focus.

4. Symbolism of the Four Vedas & Life Stages: The four rounds can represent the four Vedas (Rig, Yajur, Sama, Atharva) or the four stages of life in Hindu philosophy (Brahmacharya, Grihastha, Vanaprastha, and Sannyasa), reinforcing its spiritual depth.

The Daily Ritual of Sun Salutations

Surya Namaskar is not just a physical practice but a moving meditation, a prayer to the cosmic sun within. With four rounds each morning, you harness your inner fire, establish resilience, and create a foundation for self-discipline. Whether you are a beginner or an advanced practitioner, this sequence will bring harmony, strength, and renewed purpose to your daily life. Let every breath be an offering, every movement a devotion, and every practice a step toward self-realization.

Completing four rounds would mean you have flowed through a total of 48 steps in your practice. That amounts to a total of 40 asanas not accounting for the first and last step in each round.

We are reminded us to awaken all our senses, just as the Sun Salutations awaken the body and mind. Through this practice, we cultivate clarity, vitality, and the ability to perceive life's beauty with wisdom.

Rise. Shine. Repeat.

Chapter 11:

The 3 Minutes of Stillness – Shavasana as a Gateway to Deep Restoration

Shloka:
शान्तिः शान्तिः शान्तिः ॥
(Śāntiḥ śāntiḥ śāntiḥ.)

Translation:
"Peace, peace, peace."

Source: Vedic Chanting Tradition

Shavasana cultivates deep restoration, reinforcing SHIVA's emphasis on stillness. Shavasana, or the Corpse Pose, is often dismissed as a mere resting posture at the end of yoga practice. However, to those who understand its true depth, Shavasana is the gateway to profound mental, physical, and spiritual restoration. It is in this sacred stillness that transformation occurs—where the boundaries between the body and the infinite dissolve. This act of complete surrender mirrors Lord Shiva himself—the Adiyogi, who embodies both the ultimate stillness and the infinite potential of existence.

Shavasana and Shiva: The Dance of Stillness and Awakening

Shiva, in his form as Mahadeva, is often depicted as lying in deep yogic meditation, utterly still, yet infinitely powerful. His stillness is not mere inactivity but a potent energy, a deep presence that transcends the material world. Shavasana invites us to embody this same energy—to cultivate the art of doing nothing while allowing everything within us to settle, integrate, and renew.

In the yogic tradition, death is not seen as an end but as a transition. Shavasana, named after the corpse, symbolizes this transition—not a literal death but a metaphorical release of old patterns, stress, and accumulated fatigue. It is a moment where we let go, trust, and allow our consciousness to expand beyond the physical body.

The Science Behind Shavasana: Rest, Recover, Rejuvenate

While Shavasana holds immense spiritual significance, it is also scientifically backed as one of the most beneficial postures for the nervous system. By consciously relaxing in stillness, the body shifts from the sympathetic nervous system (fight-or-flight mode) into the parasympathetic nervous system (rest-and-digest mode).

Here's how it benefits different systems of the body:

1. The Nervous System – Calming Effect

- Reduces cortisol and adrenaline levels, counteracting stress.
- Lowers blood pressure and slows heart rate, inducing deep relaxation.
- Enhances neuroplasticity, allowing the brain to rewire itself for positivity.

2. The Musculoskeletal System – Releasing Tension

- Provides deep muscular relaxation, reducing chronic tension.
- Enhances circulation, promoting muscle recovery and flexibility.
- Improves posture by aligning the spine in a neutral position.

3. The Respiratory System – Expanding Breath Awareness

- Encourages diaphragmatic breathing, increasing oxygen exchange.
- Improves lung capacity over time by reducing habitual breath-holding patterns.

4. The Endocrine System – Hormonal Balance

- Balances hormones responsible for mood regulation, such as serotonin and dopamine.
- Improves sleep by enhancing melatonin production.

5. The Mind – Pathway to Meditation

- Cultivates mindfulness by bringing awareness to the present moment.
- Acts as a natural entry point to meditation, reducing mental chatter.
- Enhances focus and creativity by allowing the mind to rest and reset.

The Power of 3 Minutes: Why This Duration?

Many practitioners believe that Shavasana should last at least 10 minutes to fully integrate the benefits of yoga practice. While longer durations are ideal, even a simple 3-minute Shavasana can be profoundly effective when practiced daily. The number three holds deep spiritual significance—it represents creation, preservation, and destruction, the three fundamental aspects of Shiva's cosmic dance (Trimurti). In just three minutes of stillness, we experience:

1. Grounding – A reconnection with our breath and body.
2. Integration – A merging of movement and stillness.
3. Renewal – A reset of the nervous system.

When practiced consistently, this short yet potent stillness rewires the brain, making calmness a default state rather than a fleeting experience.

How to Practice Shavasana Effectively

Step 1: Set Up Your Space

- Lie flat on your back, allowing your legs to relax and fall naturally apart.
- Place your arms slightly away from your body, palms facing upward in a gesture of receptivity.
- Close your eyes gently and let your facial muscles relax completely.

Step 2: Scan the Body

- Mentally scan from the toes to the crown of your head, softening each part.
- Let go of any tension or gripping sensation.

Step 3: Focus on the Breath

- Allow your breath to flow naturally, without force.
- Observe each inhalation and exhalation, cultivating a state of detached awareness.

Step 4: Enter Deep Stillness

- If thoughts arise, acknowledge them and let them pass like clouds in the sky.
- Focus on the sensation of simply being—without doing, analyzing, or striving.

Step 5: Emerging from Stillness

- Slowly bring awareness back to the body.
- Wiggle the fingers and toes, deepen the breath, and roll to one side before sitting up.
- Take a moment of gratitude before moving forward with your day.

Integrating Shavasana into Daily Life

While Shavasana is often practiced at the end of a yoga session, its benefits extend beyond the mat. In our fast-paced, overstimulated world, moments of stillness are essential. Consider integrating Shavasana:

- Before sleep – A quick reset for deep rest.
- During work breaks – A 3-minute desk relaxation to restore focus.
- After intense conversations – To re-center and respond rather than react.

By consciously embracing stillness, we become more present, more patient, and more powerful in our daily interactions.

The Stillness of Shiva, The Stillness Within

In the stillness of Shavasana, we meet the essence of Shiva—the infinite silence behind all movement, the eternal witness of existence. When we cultivate this daily practice, we do not merely rest; we reconnect with our own divine nature. In that space of surrender, the chaos of life finds its rhythm, and the soul, like Shiva in deep meditation, discovers its boundless peace.

Be still, be whole.

Chapter 12

The 2 Vibrational Chants

Mantras for Mental Clarity and Balance

Shloka:

नादोपासनया ब्रह्माणं समुपासते ।

(Nādo-pāsanayā brahmāṇaṁ samupāsate.)

Translation:

"Through sound meditation,
One attains the essence of Brahman."

Source: Nada Bindu Upanishad

Chanting aligns one's vibration with universal consciousness. Chanting is a bridge between movement and stillness, sound and silence, the material and the divine. The 5-4-3-2-1 Method includes two vibrational chants as a crucial step toward inner harmony, mental clarity, and energetic balance. In this practice, chanting is not simply a vocal exercise but a method of tuning into the cosmic vibration, aligning the body and mind with universal consciousness.

While any two mantras or sacred words can be chosen for this practice, one of the most powerful and universal sounds to chant is Om (Aum). In the 5-4-3-2-1 Method, it is chanted once at the beginning of practice and once at the end, serving as both an invocation and a closure to the session.

For practitioners of other faiths or those who prefer non-religious options, alternative chants and affirmations are also provided.

Om: The Primordial Sound

Om (Aum) is considered the sound of creation, the vibration that underlies all existence. It is the most sacred mantra in Hinduism, Buddhism, and Jainism, representing the union of the physical, mental, and spiritual dimensions.

The syllable Aum is composed of three distinct sounds:

1. "A" (Ahh) – Represents creation, the waking state (Jagrat), and the physical world.
2. "U" (Ooo) – Represents preservation, the dream state (Swapna), and the mental realm.
3. "M" (Mmm) – Represents dissolution, the deep sleep state (Sushupti), and the spiritual domain.

Together, these three sounds merge into silence, signifying the ultimate state of enlightenment (Turiya).

The Benefits of Chanting Om

Chanting Om has been studied extensively for its physiological and psychological effects. Some of the key benefits include:

1. Mental Clarity & Focus

- Chanting Om activates the vagus nerve, helping to reduce stress and enhance cognitive function.
- It increases alertness while simultaneously inducing relaxation, making it an excellent tool for mindfulness.

2. Emotional Balance

- Om chanting is known to balance the limbic system, which regulates emotions.
- It reduces symptoms of anxiety and depression by fostering a deep sense of connection and peace.

3. Respiratory & Cardiovascular Health

- Deep, rhythmic chanting regulates breath, improving lung capacity and oxygenation.
- It lowers heart rate and blood pressure, promoting cardiovascular well-being.

4. Spiritual Connection

- Om is considered the "Nada Brahman" (cosmic sound), helping practitioners attune themselves to higher states of consciousness.

Alternative Chants

For those who wish to explore beyond Om, here are additional mantras and affirmations that align with the 5-4-3-2-1 Method. Or you can simply humm in your mind.

Hindu Mantras:

1. "So Ham" – Meaning "I am that," this mantra affirms the connection between individual and universal consciousness.
2. "Om Namah Shivaya" – A powerful mantra invoking Lord Shiva, the supreme yogi, for inner transformation.
3. "Lokah Samastah Sukhino Bhavantu" – A chant for universal peace and harmony.
4. "Gayatri Mantra" – A sacred Vedic mantra for wisdom and enlightenment.

Buddhist & Non-Hindu Chants:

1. "Om Mani Padme Hum" – A Tibetan Buddhist chant invoking compassion and wisdom.
2. "Sat Nam" – A Sikh mantra meaning "Truth is my identity."
3. "Shalom" – A Hebrew word for peace and harmony.
4. "Ameen" – An Islamic affirmation of faith and surrender.
5. "Jesus"- A Christian sacred chant

Non-Religious Affirmations:

1. "I am at peace."
2. "I am present in this moment."

How to Incorporate Chanting into Practice

In the 5-4-3-2-1 Method, two chants are used:

- At the beginning: To center the mind, invoke positive energy, and set the tone for practice.

- At the end: To integrate the experience, express gratitude, and seal the practice with serenity.

Step-by-Step Guide to Chanting Om:

1. Sit comfortably with a straight spine, either in Sukhasana (Easy Pose) or Padmasana (Lotus Pose).
2. Close your eyes and take a few deep breaths to relax.
3. Inhale deeply, and on the exhale, chant Om in a slow, sustained manner.
4. Feel the vibrations in your chest, throat, and head.
5. Repeat 3-5 times, allowing the sound to dissolve into silence.

Chanting and the Energy Centers (Chakras)

Different mantras resonate with different chakras, aligning and balancing the body's energy system:

- Om – Crown Chakra (Sahasrara) – Enlightenment
- So Ham – Third Eye Chakra (Ajna) – Intuition
- Om Mani Padme Hum – Heart Chakra (Anahata) – Compassion
- Om Namah Shivaya – Throat Chakra (Vishuddha) – Expression

By practicing mantra chanting, we open the flow of energy and elevate our state of being.

Chanting is a sacred tool for aligning with the divine, silencing mental noise, and cultivating a deep sense of balance. Whether you choose the universal Om, a traditional mantra, or a personal affirmation, the act of chanting itself is transformative. As you integrate these two sacred chants into your daily practice, feel the resonance within and allow it to guide you toward clarity, peace, and self-discovery.

Chant. Elevate. Transcend.

Chapter 13

The 1 Powerful Intention – Setting the Tone for Success and Serenity

Shloka:

सङ्कल्पमूलं आत्मनो बन्धमोक्षौ भवतः ।।

(Saṅkalpamūlaṁ ātmano bandhamokṣau bhavataḥ.)

Translation:

"Intention is the root of both bondage and liberation."

Source: Yoga Vasistha

This emphasizes the power of setting a strong intention. In the SHIVA framework, a clear and focused sankalpa (intention) directs the mind and energy towards transformation.

The Sacred Power of Intention (Sankalpa)

In the grand cosmic dance of Shiva, every movement, every breath, and every sound carries purpose. Intention, or *Sankalpa,* is the silent yet profound force that directs the energy of our actions. Just as Lord Shiva's meditative stillness holds the blueprint of the universe, our intentions shape our personal and professional realities.

In the 5-4-3-2-1 methodology, we conclude each practice by setting a powerful intention. This single act, though seemingly simple, holds the potential to realign our thoughts, actions, and energy toward success, clarity, and peace.

Why Set an Intention?

An intention is more than a goal; it is a deep, heartfelt commitment to a way of being. Unlike fleeting desires, an intention is rooted in the present moment. When reinforced through movement, breathwork, and meditation, it becomes a powerful tool for transformation.

Modern science confirms what ancient yogis knew intuitively: the mind's focus shapes reality. Neurological studies suggest that setting an intention activates the reticular activating system (RAS) in the brain, filtering perceptions and decisions to align with the chosen focus. This is why people who set clear intentions often experience profound shifts in their external and internal worlds.

Intention vs. Goal: Understanding the Difference

While goals are necessary, intentions give them meaning. When you set an intention before your yoga and meditation practice, you infuse your actions with deeper purpose and direction.

Intention	Goal
Focuses on the present moment	Focuses on the future
Internal transformation	External achievement
Aligned with emotions and values	Based on results and milestones
Rooted in mindfulness and self-awareness	Requires action steps and tracking

The Psychological Benefits of Setting Intentions

1. Enhances Mental Clarity: By defining what truly matters, intentions cut through mental clutter.
2. Reduces Stress and Anxiety: A clear intention aligns emotions, reducing overthinking and doubt.
3. Strengthens Willpower: Reaffirming an intention daily rewires the brain for resilience.
4. Improves Decision-Making: When guided by a strong Sankalpa, choices become clearer and more aligned with personal truth.
5. Promotes a Sense of Purpose: Whether in corporate life or personal life, intentions create direction and meaning.

Crafting Your Personal Intention

A strong intention should be simple, present-tense, and emotionally charged. Here are key steps to creating one:

1. Reflect: Ask yourself what quality or feeling you want to cultivate.
2. Condense: Keep it short and powerful.
3. State it Positively: Instead of "I will not doubt myself," say, "I trust in my abilities."
4. Feel It: Visualize and emotionally connect with your intention.
5. Repeat Daily: Reinforce it through breathwork, meditation, and yoga.

Powerful Intention Statements for Different Aspects of Life Corporate Life

- "I communicate with confidence and clarity."
- "I lead with wisdom and integrity."
- "I remain calm and centered in high-pressure situations."
- "I welcome challenges as opportunities for growth."
- "I trust in my skills and the value I bring."
- "I navigate office politics with grace and authenticity."
- "I embrace change and adapt with resilience."
- "My work aligns with my higher purpose."

Powerful Intention Statements for Personal Growth and Well-Being

- "I am grounded, present, and at peace."
- "I nourish my body and mind with love and care."
- "I release what no longer serves me."
- "I welcome abundance and joy into my life."
- "I forgive myself and others with an open heart."
- "I cultivate patience and understanding."
- "I live in alignment with my highest self."

Powerful Intention Statements for Parenting

- "I nurture my child with love, patience, and understanding."
- "I lead with compassion and respond with kindness."
- "I embrace each moment with my child as an opportunity to grow together."
- "I listen deeply and respond with wisdom and empathy."
- "I create a safe and loving space for my child to express themselves."
- "I balance guidance with trust, allowing my child to flourish."
- "I release perfection and embrace the beauty of learning alongside my child."
- "I stay present and engaged, giving my child the attention they deserve."
- "I cultivate patience and meet challenges with a calm heart."
- "I honor my child's individuality and support their unique path."
- "I model the values I wish to instill in my child through my actions."

The Connection Between Intention, Asanas, and Breathwork

1. Asanas (Physical Postures)
    - Movement makes the body receptive to intention. Each pose embodies a symbolic energy. For example:
        - *Vrikshasana (Tree Pose)* → Strengthens resolve.
        - *Tadasana (Mountain Pose)* → Instills confidence.
        - *Shavasana (Corpse Pose)* → Grounds the intention into the subconscious.
2. Breathwork (Pranayama)
    - The breath is a bridge between the conscious and subconscious mind. Intentions set during mindful breathing penetrate deeper into awareness.
    - *Nadi Shodhana (Alternate Nostril Breathing)* helps calm the mind before setting an intention.
    - *Bhastrika (Bellows Breath)* energizes the body and reinforces focus.

3. Meditation (Dhyana)
    - A quiet mind receives and amplifies the power of intention.
    - Mantra meditation with affirmations strengthens the intention's vibrational frequency.
    - A simple practice: Sit in stillness, inhale deeply, mentally repeat the intention, exhale, and release doubt.

The Transformative Impact of Daily Intentions

Practicing the 5-4-3-2-1 Method with a strong intention sets a clear course for personal and professional transformation. When applied consistently:

- Self-doubt diminishes as the mind aligns with its higher purpose.
- Workplace interactions improve with mindful communication and emotional intelligence.
- Daily stress becomes manageable, leading to better decision-making and creativity.
- Life feels more fulfilling as clarity replaces confusion.

In the vast cosmic play orchestrated by Lord Shiva, intention is the thread that weaves together movement, breath, and stillness. It is the silent whisper that shapes destiny. Whether you seek success in your career, harmony in your relationships, or inner serenity, let your intentions be the guiding light on your path.

As you step onto your mat and into your daily life, remember: Every thought you choose, every breath you take, and every step you move forward shapes your reality. Set your intention. Live with purpose. And let your journey toward success and serenity begin.

One thought, infinite power.

Part 3:

Mastering the Shiva Mindset and Walking the Lifelong Shiva Path

Shloka:
श्रद्धावान् लभते ज्ञानं तत्परः संयतेन्द्रियः ।
(Śraddhāvān labhate jñānaṁ tatparaḥ saṁyatendriyaḥ.)

Translation:
"The one with faith, dedication, and self-control attains wisdom."

Source: Bhagavad Gita (4.39)

This verse underscores the lifelong discipline of the SHIVA path, where persistence, self-regulation, and deep trust in the practice lead to ultimate transformation.

Shiva is more than a deity—he is an eternal state of being. He represents the mind that is unshaken, the heart that is boundless, and the soul that is fearless. To walk the lifelong path of Shiva is to cultivate awareness, resilience, and detachment, balancing the demands of the external world with the stillness of inner truth.

The Shiva Mindset is not about renunciation in the traditional sense—it is about mastery of the self while fully engaging with life's responsibilities. Whether you are a corporate leader, an entrepreneur, a parent, a seeker, or a warrior on the battlefield of modern life, embodying Shiva's essence can transform the way you think, act, and evolve.

This section explores the connection between the philosophical SHIVA technique and the practical 5-4-3-2-1 practice in action by bringing it all together to help us truly transform into effective leaders, mindful partners and parents,, and fulfilled individuals.

The Three Pillars of the Shiva Mindset

Shiva's life offers a blueprint for success and serenity:

- He is the ultimate Yogi, immersed in deep meditation, yet he is also the fierce warrior who destroys ignorance.
- He is the ideal husband, devoted to Parvati, yet he is also the cosmic wanderer, free from attachment.
- He is the compassionate protector, shielding devotees, yet he is also the ascetic, drinking poison for the welfare of the world.

To master the Shiva mindset is to embrace these paradoxes. It is to cultivate the ability to act without ego, love without attachment, lead without fear, and surrender without weakness. It is the ability to work with unwavering focus, make decisions with clarity and wisdom, and embrace both stillness and dynamism in perfect balance.

1. Tapas – The Fire of Discipline

Shiva's unwavering meditation symbolizes the power of one-pointed focus. Whether on the yoga mat, in the boardroom, or at home, discipline is the foundation of mastery. A strong daily practice of movement, breath, and meditation sharpens both the mind and body, ensuring that challenges do not disturb inner peace.

Shiva Mindset Lesson: Cultivate inner discipline through structured habits, daily self-reflection, and resilience in adversity.

2. Vairagya – The Art of Detached Involvement

Shiva teaches the balance between total engagement and total detachment. He fights battles but remains untouched by victory or defeat. He loves deeply but is not bound by attachment. True success is not about clinging—it is about flowing.

Shiva Mindset Lesson: Engage fully in life's roles—leader, parent, partner—but do not let identity consume you. Work hard, love deeply, but remain centered.

3. Anandam – The Bliss of Being

Shiva is both the silent yogi and the ecstatic dancer (Nataraja). Life is not just about discipline and detachment—it is also about joy, rhythm, and celebration. When the mind is free, even challenges become part of the dance.

Shiva Mindset Lesson: Do not take life too seriously. Practice gratitude, humor, and lightness, knowing that life itself is a play of energy.

The Lifelong Shiva Path – A Daily Practice of Living with Purpose

Mastering the Shiva mindset is not about following rituals alone—it is about embodying a way of thinking, acting, and being. The 54321 methodology, combined with deep self-inquiry, ensures that every day becomes a step toward clarity, strength, and freedom.

1. Move with Purpose (Asanas) – Strengthen the body, sharpen the mind.
2. Breathe with Awareness (Pranayama) – Control energy, control destiny.
3. Sit in Stillness (Meditation) – Find answers within, not outside.
4. Speak with Intention (Mantras & Affirmations) – Words create reality.
5. Act with Clarity (Dharma & Intention-Setting) – Live with unwavering purpose.

To walk the Shiva path is to integrate strength with surrender, wisdom with action, and detachment with love. It is a path of fearless authenticity, where success is not measured by external achievements alone but by inner mastery.

Shiva is already within you—this journey is simply about remembering.

Om Namah Shivaya.

Chapter 14

Creating Your SHIVA Space

Shloka:

शुद्धेऽन्तःकरणे योगी देशे काले च तत्परः ।

(Śuddhe'ntaḥkaraṇe yogī deśe kāle ca tatparaḥ.)

Translation:

"A yogi, with a pure mind, must practice in a sacred space and time."

Source: Hatha Yoga Pradipika (1.12)

This highlights the importance of creating a dedicated, serene, and spiritually uplifting environment for SHIVA practice. A sacred space amplifies energy and enhances focus.

The Three Elements of a Sacred SHIVA Space

Every great transformation requires a sacred space—a place where the mind finds clarity, the body finds alignment, and the spirit finds peace. Whether in the Himalayas, an ancient temple, or deep within meditation, Shiva's presence is always rooted in sacred stillness. To integrate the SHIVA technique into daily life, we must create an intentional space that supports practice, reflection, and growth.

1. Physical Space: Design for Energy and Focus

The environment where you practice affects the depth and consistency of your discipline. Whether in your home, office, or outdoors, set up a space that supports body-mind alignment.

- Choose a Dedicated Spot: Even if small, a specific location for your practice conditions the mind to enter a meditative state faster.
- Keep it Clean and Uncluttered: A clear space fosters a clear mind. Shiva's meditation ground, Mount Kailash, is vast and pure—your space should evoke similar clarity and stillness.

- Incorporate Sacred Symbols: An image of Shiva, Om, a diya (lamp), rudraksha beads, or a simple meditation cushion can serve as an anchor for your practice.
- Use Natural Elements: Shiva represents the five elements—earth, water, fire, air, and ether. Bring these into your space through plants, a water bowl, incense, or an open window.

Tip: If you work long hours, create a portable SHIVA space with a small object—a bead, a mantra card, or a mobile app for chants. This way, your practice travels with you.

2. Mental Space: Creating an Unbreakable Routine

Even the best physical space is useless if the mind is distracted. The goal is to condition your mind to associate your SHIVA practice with calm, focus, and renewal.

- Set a Non-Negotiable Time: Decide when your practice happens each day and commit to it like a meeting with your highest self.
- Reduce Digital Disruptions: Silence notifications, set your phone to Do Not Disturb, and let others know this time is sacred.
- Use Rituals to Enter and Exit Practice: Lighting a lamp, chanting Om, or taking three deep breaths can signal the mind to shift from activity to stillness.
- Practice Gratitude Before and After: A simple "Thank you for this moment" reinforces the mental connection to discipline and devotion.

Tip: If you struggle with consistency, habit-stack your practice with something you already do—like right after waking up or before your morning coffee.

3. Energetic Space: Aligning Inner and Outer Vibration

Your inner state shapes your outer world. Shiva's presence is not just in a temple or the Himalayas—it is in your breath, your awareness, and your energy.

- Breathwork to Set Energy: Before starting, take five deep breaths to signal your nervous system to shift into practice mode.
- Mantras to Clear the Space: Chanting Om three times before practice dissolves mental noise and external distractions.

- Fire and Sound for Energy Shift: Lighting a small candle or playing soft instrumental music can elevate the vibrational frequency of the space.

Tip: If you enter your practice feeling sluggish or stressed, try a quick pranayama reset—inhale deeply, hold for a moment, and exhale slowly for five breaths.

The Power of Space in Transformation

Shiva embodies both wild nature and deep stillness. He meditates on the mountaintop but also dances as Nataraja, the cosmic force of transformation. Your SHIVA space should reflect both aspects: a place of calm retreat and a place where energy flows freely.

You don't need a perfect room to practice; what matters is intentional energy. If you cultivate discipline in your space, it spills over into every aspect of life.

1. At Home: Create a meditation corner with a small mat and a candle.
2. At Work: Use a 2-minute breathing break or silent mantra repetition to reset.
3. While Traveling: Carry a sacred object—a bead, mala, or a mantra recording—to reconnect with your practice anywhere.

The goal is not just to practice yoga but to live it. Once your SHIVA space is established, your mind and body will automatically align, making your daily practice effortless and transformative.

Key Takeaways

✅ A dedicated space enhances consistency and depth of practice.
✅ Clear physical, mental, and energetic spaces help sustain discipline.
✅ Simple rituals—breath, mantras, and symbols—anchor your practice.
✅ Your SHIVA space is not just a place—it is a mindset that travels with you.

Sacred space, sacred self.

Chapter 15

The Daily Ritual of SHIVA – 30 Minutes Each Day

Shloka:
नित्यं योगस्य साधनं भवेत् ।
(Nityaṁ yogasya sādhanam bhavet.)

Translation:
"A dedicated daily practice is the key to mastery in yoga."

Source: Shiva Samhita

SHIVA's structured yet flexible daily ritual (5-4-3-2-1) brings consistency, making self-transformation a daily habit.

The Power of a Daily Ritual

The difference between sporadic spiritual practice and true transformation lies in consistency. A ritual is not merely a routine—it is a sacred commitment to aligning body, mind, and spirit every single day.

The SHIVA framework simplifies yogic wisdom into an easy-to-follow, 30-minute daily practice using the 5-4-3-2-1 method. This ensures that every essential element—movement, breath, stillness, vibration, and intention—is seamlessly incorporated into daily life.

Just as Lord Shiva balances destruction and creation through his cosmic dance, this ritual brings a perfect balance of movement, breath, and mindfulness into your day.

The 30-Minute SHIVA Practice: A Step-by-Step Breakdown

The 5-4-3-2-1 Method is a revolutionary approach to wellness that simplifies yoga and meditation into a manageable, 30-minute daily practice. Its brilliance lies in its structure—five components that work together to create a holistic mind-body workout. Designed for accessibility and consistency, this method ensures that even the busiest professionals can reap the benefits of physical fitness, mental clarity, and emotional balance.

A detailed structure is presented in Appendix 1 as additional quick reference.

Step	Element	Duration	Purpose
5	**Sacred Movements (Asanas)**	**8-10 minutes**	**Align body and mind**
4	**Sun Salutations (Suryanamaskar)**	**8-10 minutes**	**Energize and awaken**
3	**Minutes of Stillness (Shavasana)**	**3+ minutes**	**Restore and integrate**
2	**Vibrational Chants (Mantras)**	**5-7 minutes**	**Center the mind with breathwork**
1	**Powerful Intention**	**5-7 minutes**	**Set the tone for success and serenity combined with breathwork**

The Structure of the 5-4-3-2-1 Method

The 5-4-3-2-1 Method is built on five distinct elements, each playing a crucial role in achieving a well-rounded and impactful practice:

1. 5 Asanas:
   The session begins with five foundational yoga poses, or asanas, that target key areas of the body. These poses are chosen to enhance flexibility, build strength, and improve posture. By starting with asanas, you prepare your body for the movements to come, creating a strong foundation for the rest of the practice.

2. 4 Sun Salutations:
   Following the asanas, you flow through four rounds of Sun Salutations (Surya Namaskar). This dynamic sequence is designed to synchronize breath with movement, energizing the body and promoting circulation. Sun Salutations are often referred to as the "heartbeat" of yoga because they bring vitality and rhythm to your practice.

3. 3 Minutes of Shavasana:
   After the physical exertion, the practice transitions to stillness with three minutes of Shavasana, or corpse pose. This is a restorative posture where you lie flat on your back, allowing your body to absorb the benefits of the session. It's a moment of deep relaxation, helping to reset your nervous system and promote a sense of calm.

4. 2 Chants:
   The next step involves reciting two simple yet powerful chants. Chanting creates vibrational harmony, quiets the mind, and enhances focus. These sounds are more than words—they're tools for centering yourself and connecting with your inner self.

5. 1 Intention:
   The practice concludes with setting a meaningful intention. This guiding thought or affirmation serves as a compass for your day, helping you align your actions with your values and goals.

Why the 5-4-3-2-1 Method Works

The success of the 5-4-3-2-1 Method lies in its ability to deliver maximum benefits within a short timeframe. Each component is carefully designed to address different aspects of wellness, creating a practice that is both efficient and transformative.

1. Time-Efficient:
   In just 30 minutes, you can complete a practice that touches on physical, mental, and emotional well-being. This makes it ideal for those with demanding schedules.

2. Comprehensive:
   Unlike practices that focus solely on one aspect of wellness, the 5-4-3-2-1 Method offers a balanced approach. The combination of movement, stillness, sound, and intention ensures that you address your entire being.

3. Accessible:
   The method is suitable for all levels, from beginners to experienced practitioners. Modifications can be made to suit individual needs, ensuring that everyone can participate and benefit.

4. Consistent:
   The structured format of the 5-4-3-2-1 Method makes it easy to incorporate into your daily routine. The predictability of the sequence fosters habit formation, turning wellness into a non-negotiable part of your day.

A Daily Practice That Fits Your Life

One of the most appealing aspects of the 5-4-3-2-1 Method is its adaptability. Whether you're at home, traveling, or in the office, this practice can be performed virtually anywhere. All you need is a quiet space and 30 minutes of uninterrupted time.

This flexibility makes the method accessible to a wide range of individuals. Whether you're a working parent, a frequent traveler, or someone navigating a demanding career, the 5-4-3-2-1 Method offers a solution that fits seamlessly into your lifestyle.

Step 1: The 5 Sacred Movements (8-10 minutes)

Your practice begins with five carefully selected asanas to promote flexibility, strength, and balance. These include standing, seated, all-fours, supine, and prone poses, ensuring a full-body activation.

Choose any five poses from Chapter 10 based on how you feel that day. Modify as needed, but always aim for a balance between grounding and expansion and all poses of the body from standing to supine.

Step 2: The 4 Sun Salutations (8-10 minutes)

Four rounds of Surya Namaskar (12 steps each) offer the perfect cardiovascular boost, improve circulation, and align breath with movement.

Each round is dedicated to a different aspect of holistic well-being:

1. First Round – Physical body: Activate muscles and joints
2. Second Round – Breath: Sync movement with inhalation and exhalation
3. Third Round – Mind: Develop mindfulness in motion
4. Fourth Round – Energy: Feel the prana (life force) expanding

Step 3: Three Minutes of Stillness (3+ minutes)

After the dynamic flow of Sun Salutations, the body enters Shavasana for deep relaxation. This brief yet profound pause allows your body to absorb the benefits of movement, just as Lord Shiva enters deep meditation after his cosmic dance.

Step 4: Two Vibrational Chants (5 minutes)

Chanting two powerful mantras enhances mental clarity and emotional balance. You can choose from:

- Om (ॐ) – The universal vibration, aligning mind and cosmos
- Om Namah Shivaya (ॐ नमः शिवाय) – A surrender to the higher self
- So Ham (सोऽहम्) – "I am that" – A reminder of oneness
- Just hmm away as an option at the beginning and end of the session

Chanting at the beginning and end of practice creates a sacred sound bridge, connecting the external world to the inner self.

Step 5: One Powerful Intention (4 minutes)

The final step is setting one clear intention for the day ahead. It can be a simple phrase, such as ones below or choose from the ones provided in chapter 13.

"I am centered and strong in all situations."
"I bring clarity and wisdom to my work today."
"I approach every challenge with grace and strength."

Pairing this intention with breath and visualization makes it even more effective.

Key Takeaways

✅ **A structured 30-minute SHIVA practice combines movement, breath, stillness, vibration, and intention.**
✅ **The 5-4-3-2-1 method ensures a holistic approach to well-being.**
✅ **Consistency is the key—daily practice leads to deep transformation.**

Consistency builds mastery.

Chapter 16

Practical Application in High-Performance Work Environments and Personal Life

Shloka:

योगः कर्मसु कौशलम् ।।

(Yogaḥ karmasu kauśalam.)

Translation:

"Yoga is skill in action."

Source: Bhagavad Gita (2.50)

The SHIVA framework enhances productivity and clarity in professional and personal life.

Why SHIVA Matters in Work and Life

Shiva represents balance between action and stillness, discipline and detachment, creation and dissolution. These same principles apply to high-performance workplaces and personal success.

Corporate leaders, executives, and professionals often struggle with stress, decision fatigue, and burnout. The SHIVA framework provides a structured approach to maintaining clarity, efficiency, and emotional intelligence in demanding environments.

Integrating SHIVA in the Workplace

1. The Power of Intention in Leadership

- Start the day with a clear intention statement before meetings or presentations.
- Use breath awareness before making major decisions to ensure clarity.
- Apply the detachment principle—take right action without attachment to results.

Example: Before entering a negotiation, take three deep breaths, set the intention, "I communicate with clarity and confidence," and proceed with calm focus.

2. Using Breathwork for Stress Management

- Take one-minute breathing breaks between tasks to reset focus.
- Use 4-7-8 breathing before high-stakes meetings. For this technique, breathe in for a count of 4 seconds, hold the breath in for a count of 7 seconds and then breathe out for a count of 8 seconds. You can simply count up in your mind or use a timer.
- Try pranayama at your desk to avoid workplace burnout.

Tip: If overwhelmed, pause for five deep breaths, mentally repeating "I am in control of my energy."

3. Applying Movement and Stillness in the Office

- Stretch for five minutes every two hours to prevent stiffness.
- If possible, practice a few rounds of Surya Namaskar before work to boost morning energy.
- End the day with Shavasana or mindfulness meditation to transition from work to personal life.

Tip: A brief seated twist or gentle forward fold at your desk can release tension and improve posture.

Integrating SHIVA in Personal Life

1. Creating a SHIVA-Inspired Evening Routine

- Close your day with reflection—list three things you are grateful for.
- End with stillness—spend three minutes in silence before bed.
- Use mantras for deep rest—softly chant Om or a calming phrase.

Example: Before sleeping, say "I surrender all worries. I welcome peace."

2. Bringing SHIVA's Detachment into Relationships
   - Accept that you cannot control others—only your own reactions.
   - Respond with calm instead of impulse—pause before reacting emotionally.
   - Practice "let go" moments—release unnecessary arguments or worries.

Tip: When upset, silently repeat "I choose peace over reaction."

Key Takeaways

✅ **The SHIVA method can be seamlessly integrated into high-performance work and personal life.**
✅ **Breathwork, intention-setting, and movement enhance productivity and clarity.**
✅ **Shiva's balance of detachment and discipline is the ideal mindset for success.**

Yoga is life.

Chapter 17

Overcoming Challenges and Staying Consistent

Shloka:
नायमात्मा बलहीनेन लभ्यः ।।
(Nāyam ātmā balahīnena labhyaḥ.)

Translation:
"The Self is not attained by the weak."

Source: Mundaka Upanishad (3.2.4)

Consistency requires inner strength, perseverance, and discipline.

Introduction: The Power of Perseverance

Embracing the SHIVA Technique as part of your daily routine can be deeply transformative, yet, like any meaningful habit, it requires dedication, discipline, and adaptability. Challenges such as time constraints, lack of motivation, physical limitations, and inconsistency can arise. However, overcoming these challenges is where true growth happens.

By addressing these obstacles with intention, creativity, and self-compassion, you can create a sustainable and fulfilling practice that supports both your personal and professional life. The SHIVA Technique is not meant to be rigid; rather, it is a flexible system designed to adapt to your unique lifestyle and needs.

Let's explore the common challenges practitioners face and practical solutions to ensure you stay committed to your journey.

Common Challenges and How to Overcome Them

1. "I Don't Have Enough Time"

In today's fast-paced world, finding 30 minutes for your SHIVA practice might seem daunting. However, even the busiest professionals and parents can integrate this technique with the right mindset and time management.

Strategies to Overcome Time Constraints

- Prioritize with Purpose: Identify time-wasting activities (such as excessive social media scrolling) and replace them with SHIVA practice.
- Schedule It Like a Meeting: Treat your practice as non-negotiable—set a calendar reminder and commit to it like an important work appointment.
- Start Small, Build Gradually: If 30 minutes feels overwhelming, begin with 10 minutes and slowly increase the duration as consistency builds.
- Integrate SHIVA into Daily Life:
    - ➢ Practice standing asanas while waiting for coffee to brew.
    - ➢ Do a 3-minute breathwork session before bed.
    - ➢ Chant a mantra during your commute.

Consistency matters more than duration—a short but regular practice is far more effective than long, infrequent sessions.

2. "I Lose Motivation Easily"

It's natural for motivation to fluctuate. Some days, you will feel energized and ready to practice, while on other days, it might feel like a burden. This is where discipline takes over motivation.

Strategies to Stay Motivated

- Set Clear Goals: Do you want mental clarity, flexibility, or stress relief? Defining your "why" will anchor your practice.
- Track Your Progress: Maintain a journal to log how you feel before and after each session. Seeing improvements over time boosts motivation.
- Join a Support System: Practicing with a community fosters accountability. Connect with like-minded individuals, share your journey, and celebrate small wins together. Consider joining Ethnik Yoga's free Facebook group to keep you motivated. Scan QR code for this and other resources at the end of the book.
- Reward Yourself: Pair your practice with something enjoyable—such as a favorite herbal tea afterward or extra time in Shavasana.
- Use Visual Reminders: Place a meaningful quote, an image of Shiva, or your intention statement in your practice space for inspiration.
- Remember: Discipline sustains you when motivation fades.

3. "I Have Physical Limitations or Injuries"

Your body is unique, and physical constraints—whether due to injury, age, or flexibility levels—can make certain poses challenging. However, the SHIVA Technique is adaptable.

Strategies to Adapt Your Practice

- Modify Poses: Use props like yoga blocks, straps, or cushions to support your movements.
- Focus on Breathwork and Chanting: Even if you cannot perform advanced asanas, the benefits of pranayama and mantra chanting are profound.
- Listen to Your Body: Yoga is not about pushing through pain. Honor what feels good and modify as needed.
- Seek Guidance: If unsure, work with a yoga teacher or therapist to tailor the practice to your abilities.

The SHIVA Technique is inclusive—it welcomes all bodies and abilities.

Building Consistency: The Key to Transformation

1. Establish a Ritual

A structured ritual helps embed your practice into your daily routine.

- Set a Fixed Time & Space: Whether it's morning or evening, having a dedicated practice space creates an anchor for consistency.
- Create an Inviting Atmosphere: Light a candle, play soft chanting music, or use essential oils to mark the beginning of your session.
- Use a Habit Link: Connect your practice to an existing habit—right after brushing your teeth or before breakfast.

2. Be Flexible with Your Routine

Life is unpredictable. Instead of skipping your practice entirely, adapt it to fit your day.

- Shorten Your Session: If busy, perform just two elements (e.g., Sun Salutation + Shavasana).

- Practice Anywhere: Traveling? Do pranayama and chanting in your hotel room.
- Forgive Yourself: Missed a day? Don't quit. Restart the next day.

3. Cultivate Self-Discipline

- Discipline sustains you when excitement fades.
- Commit for 21 Days: It takes about three weeks to form a habit—challenge yourself to practice daily for 21 days.
- Visualize Your Success: Before practice, picture yourself completing it and feeling rejuvenated.

Keep Your "Why" in Mind: Constantly remind yourself why you started.

4. Celebrate Small Wins

Acknowledging progress keeps you motivated.

- Reflect on Achievements: Whether it's holding a pose longer or feeling calmer, acknowledge growth.
- Share Your Journey: Engage with a yoga group or an online forum to celebrate milestones.
- Treat Yourself: Invest in a new yoga mat or book as a reward for your dedication.

The Power of Persistence

Staying consistent with the SHIVA Technique will bring profound benefits:

- Physical: Greater strength, flexibility, and vitality.
- Mental: Increased focus, clarity, and stress resilience.
- Emotional: Deeper self-awareness and inner peace.

Every small effort compounds over time. Even on difficult days, showing up—even if only for a few minutes—keeps the momentum alive.

Remember: Shiva is the ultimate yogi—not because he never faced challenges, but because he mastered stillness amidst chaos.

Real-Life Scenarios & Solutions

Scenario 1: "I'm Too Busy Today"
✅ Solution: Commit to just 5 minutes—even deep breathing or chanting counts.

Scenario 2: "I Don't Feel Like Practicing"
✅ Solution: Start with your favorite part (e.g., a mantra or a gentle stretch)—you'll naturally want to continue.

Scenario 3: "I'm Struggling with a Pose"
✅ Solution: Modify it! Use props, adjust alignment, or substitute with a simpler pose.

Keep practicing. Your transformation is unfolding.

Show up, no matter what. Your path awaits.

Chapter 18

Closing Thoughts: Step Forward into Your SHIVA Journey

Shloka:
सर्वधर्मान्परित्यज्य मामेकं शरणं व्रज ।।
(Sarva-dharmān parityajya mām ekaṁ śaraṇaṁ vraja.)

Translation:
"Abandon all doubts and surrender fully to your path."

Source: Bhagavad Gita (18.66)

Letting go of hesitation and fully embracing the SHIVA journey leads to ultimate growth. As you close the pages of this book, I hope you feel something stirring within—perhaps a newfound sense of purpose, a desire to deepen your practice, or a simple realization that transformation is possible for you. The journey you have embarked upon is not merely about physical postures, breathwork, or meditation. It is about cultivating a way of life, a mindset, and a spiritual strength that will carry you through every challenge, decision, and triumph.

You now hold the key to a practice that can redefine how you live each day. The 5-4-3-2-1 SHIVA Method is not just a routine; it is a compass for balance, clarity, and inner power. But reading about it is only the beginning. True transformation happens when you take action.

The Next Step: Experience the methodology in a daily practice live via Zoon

Yoga is not meant to be practiced in isolation. It thrives in community, in shared experiences, and in the energy of like-minded individuals striving for growth and self-discovery. That's why I invite you to take this practice off the page and into your life—starting today.

At Ethnik Yoga and Arva Yoga, we are building a space where individuals from all backgrounds—whether beginner or advanced—can come together to experience the power of structured, mindful, and practical yoga. It's a place where the ancient meets the modern, where tradition meets innovation, and where you can experience the depth of yoga's age-old wisdom through movement, breath, and stillness.

What Awaits You?

- JOIN A CLASS – Experience the 5-4-3-2-1 SHIVA Method in action with a guided session that integrates asanas, pranayama, chanting, and meditation.
- LIVE ONLINE SESSIONS – Practice from the comfort of your home with structured classes designed for busy professionals, parents, and seekers.
- PERSONALIZED GUIDANCE – Get direct feedback, modifications, and support from an experienced teacher to make your practice effective.
- COMMUNITY SUPPORT – Connect with a global community of individuals on the same journey, supporting and motivating each other.
- RESOURCES & LEARNING – Gain access to exclusive content, detailed explanations, and continued guidance beyond this book.

Why Now? Why You?

You are here for a reason. Something inside you called you to this book, to Shiva, to yoga. Perhaps you have been looking for stability amidst chaos, for strength amidst uncertainty, or for a path that aligns with your deeper self. Whatever your reason, trust that this is your moment.

You do not have to navigate this alone. The SHIVA practice is a gift meant to be experienced, refined, and shared. So why wait? Take the first step. Show up for yourself. Commit to your growth.

Visit EthnikYoga.com now and sign up for free resources today. Or scan the QR code below to get started. This is not just another yoga session. This is the beginning of your transformation. I look forward to practicing with you, guiding you, and witnessing your journey unfold.

Om Namah Shivaya! Har Har Mahadev!

With gratitude,
Vaibhavi Haridas
Founder, Ethnik Yoga & Arva Yoga

Appendix 1- 21-Day SHIVA Asana Practice Plan

Each day, commit to a 30-minute practice designed to strengthen, align, and restore your body and mind. This structured approach blends movement, breath, and intention to create a holistic transformation over three weeks.

Daily Practice Structure following 5-4-3-2-1 method (30 Minutes)

1. Opening Ritual (3-5 Minutes)
    - Arrive on your mat and take a moment to ground yourself in a seated pose of your choice.
    - Observe your breath, allowing your mind to settle.
    - Silently repeat your intention and chant one mantra to align with your purpose. You may choose to keep the same intention statement for all 21 days and use OM as your mantra, allowing for a simple yet profound practice that deepens with each session
    - Begin with gentle movements to warm up your body for Sun Salutations.
2. Sun Salutations (8-10 Minutes)
    - Flow through 4 rounds of Surya Namaskar, synchronizing breath with movement.
    - Focus on stability, breath control, and inner awareness as you awaken your energy.
3. Asana Practice (8-10 Minutes)
    - Practice 5-8 asanas, flowing mindfully, and progressing from:
        - Standing poses (strength and balance)
        - Seated poses (grounding and flexibility)
        - Quadruped poses (core activation and spinal mobility)
        - Prone poses (strength and expansion)
        - Supine poses (relaxation and integration)

- A list of simple asanas is provided in the table below but feel free to use the tracker in Appendix 2 to plan your own asanas for each day,

4. Shavasana (3+ Minutes)

   - Lie down and surrender into stillness, absorbing the effects of your practice.

   - Stay here for at least 3 minutes—or longer if needed.

5. Closing Ritual (3 Minutes)

   - Gently return to a seated position.

   - Observe your breath and reflect on your practice.

   - Silently recite your intention and chant one mantra to seal your session with purpose.

Sample Plan of Asanas for 21 days

Day	Asana Sequence	Benefits & Theme
Day 1 – Foundation of Strength	Tadasana, Sukhasana, Marjariasana, Pavanamuktasana, Bhujangasana	Builds balance, core strength, and flexibility
Day 2 – Flowing with Grace	Virabhadrasana I, Vajrasana, Balasana, Setu Bandhasana, Salabhasana	Enhances stability, digestion, and spinal flexibility
Day 3 – Awakening Vital Energy	Trikonasana, Padmasana, Vyaghrasana, Supta Matsyendrasana, Dhanurasana	Stimulates energy flow, spinal mobility, and detoxification
Day 4 – Rooted in Stability	Utkatasana, Siddhasana, Adho Mukha Svanasana, Viparita Karani, Makarasana	Strengthens legs, calms the mind, and enhances circulation
Day 5 – Centering the Mind & Body	Vrikshasana, Baddha Konasana, Parighasana, Supta Baddha Konasana, Bhujangasana	Improves focus, opens hips, and relieves lower back tension

Day	Asana Sequence	Benefits & Theme
Day 6 – Warrior's Resilience	Virabhadrasana II, Gomukhasana, Utthita Balasana, Jathara Parivartanasana, Salabhasana	Enhances endurance, opens shoulders, and strengthens the back
Day 7 – Shiva's Stillness	Samasthiti, Sukhasana, Marjariasana, Savasana, Makarasana	A deep restorative practice to reset and recharge
Day 8 – Expansion & Strength	Parsvakonasana, Vajrasana, Parighasana, Supta Matsyendrasana, Bhujangasana	Expands lung capacity, strengthens legs, and supports spinal health
Day 9 – Harnessing Inner Fire	Virabhadrasana III, Siddhasana, Vyaghrasana, Supta Baddha Konasana, Dhanurasana	Builds core strength, balance, and enhances digestion
Day 10 – Flowing Like Water	Anjaneyasana, Padmasana, Balasana, Setu Bandhasana, Salabhasana	Opens the hips, improves flexibility, and relieves stress
Day 11 – Grounding & Stability	Malasana, Baddha Konasana, Adho Mukha Svanasana, Viparita Karani, Makarasana	Deep hip opening, balances energy, and supports circulation
Day 12 – Rising with Determination	Utkatasana, Vajrasana, Marjariasana, Jathara Parivartanasana, Bhujangasana	Strengthens legs, activates digestion, and enhances spinal mobility
Day 13 – Wisdom & Intuition	Tadasana, Siddhasana, Parighasana, Supta Matsyendrasana, Dhanurasana	Strengthens posture, opens chest, and improves spinal health
Day 14 – Shiva's Warrior Spirit	Virabhadrasana I, Gomukhasana, Utthita Balasana, Setu Bandhasana, Salabhasana	Builds endurance, opens shoulders, and energizes the back
Day 15 – Balance & Surrender	Trikonasana, Padmasana, Vyaghrasana, Supta Baddha Konasana, Makarasana	Enhances balance, soothes the nervous system, and promotes relaxation

Day	Asana Sequence	Benefits & Theme
Day 16 – Strength from Within	Virabhadrasana II, Sukhasana, Marjariasana, Viparita Karani, Bhujangasana	Strengthens willpower, aligns breath with movement, and enhances circulation
Day 17 – The Power of Breath & Movement	Utkatasana, Siddhasana, Balasana, Jathara Parivartanasana, Salabhasana	Improves focus, spinal mobility, and inner awareness
Day 18 – Expansion & Letting Go	Parsvakonasana, Vajrasana, Parighasana, Setu Bandhasana, Bhujangasana	Improves flexibility, lung capacity, and spinal health
Day 19 – Flow into Serenity	Vrikshasana, Baddha Konasana, Vyaghrasana, Supta Matsyendrasana, Dhanurasana	Cultivates inner balance, spinal flexibility, and digestive strength
Day 20 – Strength in Stillness	Anjaneyasana, Padmasana, Marjariasana, Viparita Karani, Makarasana	Opens hips, enhances mindfulness, and promotes relaxation
Day 21 – Shiva's Eternal Flow	Tadasana, Sukhasana, Utthita Balasana, Savasana, Bhujangasana	Deep relaxation, grounding, and complete rejuvenation

Guiding Principles for Success

☑ Balance & Adaptability – Modify as needed to honor your energy levels.
☑ Breath Awareness – Let your breath guide each movement, cultivating Shiva's balance of effort and surrender.
☑ Commitment & Presence – Stay present and dedicated, trusting in the transformation this practice offers.

This three-week journey is designed to awaken your physical, mental, and spiritual potential—a path to harmony and inner mastery following the 5-4-3-2-1 method.

Om Namah Shivaya.

Appendix 2- SHIVA Method Tracker

Track your daily transformation with the SHIVA Method. Check off each element as you complete it, and reflect on your progress in the notes section. Keep one page for each day of practice by recording the date and time of your practice for that day.

5 Sacred Movements (Asanas)

- Asana 1
- Asana 2
- Asana 3
- Asana 4
- Asana 5

4 Cycles of Sun Salutations

- Sun Salutation 1
- Sun Salutation 2
- Sun Salutation 3
- Sun Salutation 4

3 Minutes of Stillness (Shavasana)

Completed Shavasana

2 Sacred Sounds (Chants at the beginning and end of the practice)

- Chant 1
- Chant 2

1 Focused Intention (Set at the beginning of the practice and mentally throughout)

Set Intention

Daily Insights & Reflection

Appendix 3- The Sacred Connection

Unlocking Shiva's Power Through the 5-4-3-2-1 Method

In this extra bonus chapter, we will explore additional connections of the methodology with SHIVA, through numerology and symbolism.

Tapping into the Divine Energy of Shiva

Shiva is more than a deity—he is the embodiment of strength, balance, and inner stillness. He is the master of yoga, meditation, and transformation, and his symbols, numbers, and practices hold deep significance for those seeking both success and inner peace.

The 5-4-3-2-1 method aligns beautifully with Shiva's principles, and by incorporating his mantras, breathwork, and visualization techniques, we can create a sacred, empowering practice that strengthens both the body and mind.

In this extra bonus section of the book, you will learn how each step of the methodology connects to Shiva's wisdom, enhancing your journey toward clarity, focus, and transformation.

SHIVA Connection to Numerology

5 – The Five Faces of Shiva (Pancha Mukha Shiva)

Shiva is often depicted with five faces, each representing a different aspect of consciousness:

1. Sadyojata (Creation & Action) – Symbolizing discipline in practice.
2. Vamadeva (Preservation & Balance) – Representing harmony in movement.
3. Aghora (Transformation & Strength) – Encouraging resilience through challenges.
4. Tatpurusha (Concentration & Meditation) – Enhancing focus and mindfulness.
5. Ishana (Liberation & Wisdom) – Awakening higher awareness.

In our practice: The 5 asanas awaken these five energies, preparing the body for strength, flexibility, and stability.

4 – The Four Arms of Shiva's Nataraja (Cosmic Dance of Life)

Shiva's Nataraja form represents the continuous cycle of life—creation, preservation, destruction, and liberation. His four arms signify:

- Drum (Damaru) – The rhythm of life, like the breath we synchronize in Sun Salutations.
- Flame (Agni) – The fire of transformation, burning away obstacles and limitations.
- Hand in Blessing (Abhaya Mudra) – Fearlessness, courage to embrace the practice.
- Foot Raised (Spiritual Ascent) – Rising beyond physical limitations to spiritual growth.

In our practice: The 4 Sun Salutations reflect this flow of transformation—moving with the breath, embracing change, and cultivating strength.

3 – Shiva's Third Eye (Wisdom & Stillness)

Shiva's third eye represents higher awareness, the ability to see beyond the physical and understand deeper truths. It is also associated with Ajna Chakra, the seat of intuition.

In our practice: The 3 minutes of Shavasana help us awaken inner wisdom, allowing the mind to quiet and experience true stillness.

Shavasana Mantra:
"Om Shanti Shanti Shanti" – Invoking peace within, around, and beyond.

2 – The Twin Forces (Ida & Pingala – Balance of Energy)

In yogic philosophy, Shiva represents the perfect balance of energies—masculine (Pingala) and feminine (Ida), action and stillness, logic and intuition. The two nostrils are associated with these energy channels, and breathwork helps harmonize them.

In our practice: The 2 chants align with the vibration of Shiva's damaru, bringing balance and healing through sacred sound.

Chants:

1. Om Namah Shivaya – *Connecting to inner strength and wisdom.*
2. Maha Mrityunjaya Mantra – *Healing, protection, and overcoming fear.*

1 – The Oneness of Consciousness (Shiva's Absolute State)

Shiva is often called Adi Yogi—the first yogi—symbolizing oneness and completeness. The third eye represents single-pointed focus, guiding us toward clarity, wisdom, and intention.

In our practice: The 1 daily intention aligns with Shiva's inner stillness, helping us stay focused on what truly matters.

Intention Mantra:
"Om Tat Purushaya Vidmahe, Mahadevaya Dhīmahi, Tanno Rudrah Prachodayāt"
(May I meditate upon the Supreme Shiva, and may he guide my thoughts toward wisdom.)

Shiva Connection to Symbolism

1. The Power of Numerology in Shiva's Symbolism

- 5 (Pancha) – Shiva is deeply associated with the number 5, representing the five elements (Pancha Mahabhutas – Earth, Water, Fire, Air, Space) and the five faces of Shiva (Panchamukha Shiva), which symbolize different aspects of consciousness.
    - This aligns with the 5 asanas in the methodology.
- 4 – Shiva holds the four Vedas in his wisdom and embodies the four stages of life (Ashramas). His four arms represent the balance between creation, preservation, destruction, and grace.
    - This connects to the 4 Sun Salutations in the practice, representing movement through these stages.

- 3 (Trinity & Trikala) – Shiva is part of the Holy Trinity (Trimurti) along with Vishnu and Brahma. He is also beyond time (Trikala - past, present, future).
    - This links to 3 minutes of Shavasana, transcending time into stillness.
- 2 (Duality & Balance) – Shiva is both the destroyer and the compassionate one, balancing opposites like masculine & feminine (Ardhanarishvara).
    - This aligns with the 2 Chants, which bring harmony between mind and spirit.
- 1 (Supreme Consciousness) – Shiva represents Oneness (Advaita), where the self merges with the universe.
    - This corresponds to the 1 Intention, which sets the mind on a singular, focused path.

2. Iconography and Symbolism in the SHIVA Technique

- Trishul (Trident - Three Forces) → Represents Shiva's control over the mind, body, and energy.
    - In the practice, this is mirrored by the 3 minutes of Shavasana, bringing all three into harmony.
- Damru (Cosmic Sound) → Symbolizes vibration, rhythm, and the sound of Om, the primal sound of the universe.
    - This is deeply connected to the 2 Chants, resonating with Shiva's divine energy.
- Third Eye (Awakening & Focus) → Represents supreme knowledge and clarity.
    - This aligns with 1 Intention, which sharpens focus for personal and professional success.
- Nataraja (Cosmic Dance) → Shiva's dance of destruction and rebirth signifies the flow of life.

    - This connects to Sun Salutations, which represent movement and transformation.

- Ganga (Divine Flow of Energy) → Flowing from Shiva's matted hair, it represents purification and renewal.
    - This symbolizes pranayama (breath work) and movement of energy in asanas.

3. Shiva's Connection to Success & Mental Peace

Shiva is not just a destroyer but also a meditator and master of inner peace. His ability to balance extreme action with deep meditation is exactly what modern professionals need—powerful action combined with stillness.

This is why the SHIVA technique and the 5-4-3-2-1 methodology is perfect—it creates a balance between:

- Physical Energy (Asanas, Sun Salutations)
- Mental Clarity (Stillness, Chanting, Intention)

By following the 5 steps daily, one aligns with Shiva's wisdom, leading to success, resilience, and serenity in both professional and personal life.

Shiva-Inspired Meditation Techniques for Professionals

To make this practice even more powerful, here are two simple Shiva-inspired meditations that can be done in just a few minutes each day:

1. Third Eye Trataka (Shiva's Vision)

- How: Light a candle and gaze at the flame. Focus your attention on the Ajna Chakra (Third Eye) while softly repeating "Om Namah Shivaya."
- Why: This awakens clarity, focus, and intuition—a crucial skill for professionals making important decisions.

2. Shiva's Breath Control (Damru Pranayama)

- How: Practice Bhramari (Bee Breath) by inhaling deeply and exhaling with a soft humming sound, resonating like Shiva's drum.
- Why: This calms the nervous system, enhances focus, and removes mental fatigue.

Bringing Shiva's Energy into Your Daily Life

By following the 5-4-3-2-1 method, you are not just performing a wellness routine—you are embodying Shiva's strength, wisdom, and stillness in every action.

- Strength (5 Asanas) – Cultivate power & resilience
- Flow (4 Sun Salutations) – Embrace transformation
- Stillness (3 Minutes Shavasana) – Awaken inner wisdom Vibration (2 Chants) – Align with cosmic energy Intention (1 Focus) – Guide your mind with clarity

No matter where you are in life, this practice grounds you, empowers you, and aligns you with Shiva's energy—helping you achieve both success and inner peace.

Shiva's Message to the Modern Professional

Shiva teaches us that balance is key—between action and stillness, ambition and surrender, strength and grace.

You don't need hours to transform your life—just 30 minutes of focused, intentional practice. And each time you practice, try to anchor your practice to an element of SHIVA! The practice will gain a new meaning!

Are you ready to embrace this sacred journey?

Om Namah Shivaya.

References

I have a personal collection of books that have inspired and helped me develop my own proprietary technique over the years. In addition to these, there are a plethora of materials – books, CDs. Manuals, study guides- that were part of my yoga teacher training courses continue to provide me with much needed insights and inspirations. It is practically impossible to list them all here but here are a few selected ones that I have learnt much from much and refer often. Mindset- Dr. Carol Dwek

1. The Upanishads- Eknath Easwaran
2. The Yogasutras of Patanjali- Sri Swami Satchidananda
3. Yoga for Mind, Body and Soul- Swami Mukundananda
4. Think and Grow Rich- Napolean Hill
5. Yoga – Alain Danielou
6. Light on Yoga and Light on Pranayama- BKS Iyengar
7. The Holy Geeta- Commentary by Swami Chinmayananda
8. The Complete Works of Swami Vivekananda
9. Kriya Yoga- Paramahansa Hariharananda

Selected Scientific Study -Yoga Effects on Brain Health: A Systematic Review of the Current Literature (https://pmc.ncbi.nlm.nih.gov/articles/PMC6971819

I have read several versions of the purana stories as well as watched hours of well-made television series Shiv Shakti episodes to really understand the nature of Shiva – and every day I learn something new!

Unlike academic texts that provide a citation for every fact, I have intentionally chosen not to include extensive references. Yoga and meditation are vast, evolving fields, with ongoing scientific research expanding our understanding every day. The purpose of this book is not to present an exhaustive academic analysis but rather to share a simple practical yoga and mindfulness technique refined through years of practical teaching—one that has consistently proven effective in real-world practice. And to anchor this practice to a supreme cause that shines in all of us- I choose to call it SHIVA!

About Vaibhavi Haridas

Vaibhavi Haridas, who often goes by Vai Haridas, is a dynamic leader with experience in technology and digital transformation, specializing in product strategy, customer-centric solutions, and operational excellence. Throughout her career, she has led large global teams, driven multimillion-dollar initiatives, and spearheaded innovative digital solutions in industries ranging from pharmaceuticals to real estate. As a senior executive, she played a pivotal role in modernizing legacy systems, optimizing business processes, and enhancing customer engagement through cutting-edge technologies. Her leadership in mergers and acquisitions, strategic growth initiatives, and platform transformations has earned her industry recognition and awards for innovation and impact.

After nearly two decades in the corporate world, Vai transitioned to her true passion—yoga and holistic wellness. A 500-hour certified yoga teacher with a specialization in meditation and Aerial Yoga, she now shares the 5-4-3-2-1 method, a unique approach to mindfulness and movement designed to help corporate professionals enhance mental clarity, reduce stress, and cultivate overall well-being. Through Arva Yoga and Ethnik Yoga, she teaches daily and weekly classes, leads transformative retreats, and conducts workshops that integrate ancient yogic wisdom with modern-day challenges.

In addition to her work in wellness, Vai is the founder of Ethnik Edge Candle Company, a brand dedicated to creating handcrafted, eco-friendly candles that blend cultural artistry with sustainable living. A portion of each sale goes toward a non-profit working in the area of child education and cancer wellness organizations.

From boardrooms to yoga studios, Vai's journey is a testament to resilience, reinvention, and the power of self-discovery. Whether leading strategic initiatives or guiding individuals on their wellness path, her mission remains the same: to empower, uplift, and transform lives—one breath at a time.

You can connect with Vai on https://www.linkedin.com/in/vaiharidas

Arva Yoga (arvayoga.org)- A 501c3 organization that offers free sessions

Ethnik Yoga Platform (ethnikyoga.com)- A virtual yoga studio

Ethnik Edge Handmade Candles and Social Entrepreneurship (ethnikedge.com)

About Arva Yoga (in words of Vaibhavi Haridas)

The year 2020 was unlike any other. The world faced unprecedented challenges, and for many, it was a time of reflection and transformation. For me, it was the year that Arva Yoga was born—a tribute to my grandmother and a mission to bring the benefits of yoga to everyone, free of charge.

The Inspiration Behind Arva Yoga- A Divine Intervention

On December 23, 2020, my paternal grandmother, Nalini Agwan, passed away. She lived a long and fulfilling life, known for her strength, courage, and generosity. She kept herself busy crafting beautiful handmade artifacts, which she joyfully gave away to family and friends. Her happiness was always tied to the happiness of others.

In our family, she was affectionately known as "Nagpur Aaji"—a name derived from her frequent travels between Nagpur and Mumbai. Despite her independence and resilience, the later years of her life were challenging. She became bedridden due to deteriorating spinal health, a condition that, while mentally alert, left her physically constrained.

Watching her decline was painful, and it led me to reflect deeply. As a dedicated yoga practitioner, I wondered: Could yoga have helped her? If she had devoted just 30 minutes a day to her well-being in her 40s or 50s, could she have avoided years of suffering? The answer, I knew, was yes. But what had stopped her? Most likely, financial constraints and a lifetime of putting others first. This realization ignited a passion within me—to share the gift of yoga freely so that no one would have to choose between their health and financial limitations.

The Meaning of Arva

The name "Arva" holds a special significance. It is a combination of the first and last letters of my children's names, symbolizing the bridge between past and future. In Latin, Arva means "fertile," representing the potential within all of us to cultivate wellness and peace. In Sanskrit, it means "fast motion wind," aligning perfectly with the graceful, free-flowing nature of aerial yoga. From traditional Hatha yoga to aerial yoga, Arva Yoga was created to offer a holistic approach to wellness, rooted in tradition yet open to innovation.

Our Mission and Growth

Arva Yoga is a unique nonprofit organization dedicated to providing free and accessible yoga classes and workshops to individuals from all walks of life. Our mission is to spread awareness of the true meaning of yoga—beyond just physical postures—to encompass mental clarity, emotional resilience, and spiritual well-being.

The challenges of 2020 highlighted not just physical health concerns but also a looming mental health crisis. As society began to recover from the COVID-19 pandemic, the need for holistic wellness became more evident than ever. Arva Yoga emerged as a beacon of hope, offering a space where people could heal, rejuvenate, and empower themselves through mindful practice.

Since its inception, Arva Yoga has grown tremendously. We have hosted hundreds of sessions and built a thriving community of over 1,200 members who regularly participate in our free classes. From weekend personal sessions to regular group practices, Arva Yoga continues to expand its reach, touching lives one soul at a time.

A Vision for the Future: Expanding the Legacy of Arva Yoga

At Arva Yoga, we envision a future where holistic wellness is not just a privilege but a way of life—accessible, transformative, and deeply rooted in both tradition and innovation. Beyond yoga classes, we are building a thriving ecosystem of wellness programs, workshops, and community-driven initiatives that nurture the mind, body, and soul. From meditation retreats to spine health workshops and movement-based therapies, Arva Yoga is evolving into a sanctuary for self-discovery, healing, and empowerment.

For me, Arva Yoga is more than an organization—it is my soul's mission and a heartfelt tribute to my grandmother's legacy. It is a bridge between the ancient wisdom of yoga and the modern need for balance, between personal well-being and collective service. Our purpose is simple yet profound: to bring health, happiness, and harmony to as many lives as possible—one mind, one body, one soul at a time.

To date, we have raised over $35,000 for women's education and social causes, and we are honored to offer a scholarship program for Yoga Teacher Training Certification—ensuring that the transformative power of yoga reaches those who need it most. But more than what we give, I feel profoundly grateful for what I receive—the privilege of connecting with like-minded, divine souls who share the same passion for service and the true essence of yoga.

A testament to this profound journey is the foreword in my book, written by Swami Atmavidyananda—an ordained monk in the Giri monastic order and Vice President of the Kriya Yoga Institute. An expert in Eastern and Western scriptures, astrology, and ancient yogic practices, Swamiji's wisdom now enriches the Arva Yoga community through monthly philosophy discourses open to all worldwide. His introduction to Arva Yoga was made possible by Shraddha Chandwadkar, our Executive Program Director, whose dedication continues to bring invaluable teachers and volunteers to our platform.

But this is just the beginning. Arva Yoga is not a solo journey—it is a collective movement. As we grow, we invite you to be part of this vision. Whether through practice, learning, or giving back, together, we can continue spreading the true meaning of yoga to every corner of the world.

Join us. Be the change. Experience the transformation.

Learn more about Arva Yoga by visiting ArvaYoga.org.

About Ethnik Yoga

Yoga is more than just movement; it is a way of life—an ancient practice that unites the mind, body, and spirit. Yet, in today's fast-paced world, yoga is often reduced to a physical workout, stripped of its deep-rooted philosophy and cultural essence. Ethnik Yoga was born out of a desire to restore the authentic wisdom of yoga while making it accessible to modern practitioners. Practices are geared toward that busy professional who wants to get a yoga session in before jumping on a Zoom call at 7:30am!

At its core, Ethnik Yoga is a sanctuary where tradition and transformation coexist. It is a space that embraces the rich heritage of yoga, integrating Sanskrit terminology, breathwork, mudras, and meditation into every session. Ethnik Yoga is a community—a place where seekers of all backgrounds come together to cultivate mindfulness, strength, and inner harmony.

Ethnik Yoga was founded in 2024 and offers authentic yoga and meditation sessions. Ethnik Yoga classes are designed to honor tradition while meeting the needs of modern practitioners. Each 45-minute session incorporates asanas, breathwork, meditation, and mindfulness—creating a holistic experience that nurtures both physical well-being and inner peace. Whether joining a live online class, participating in a retreat, or engaging in a personalized one-on-one session, students embark on a journey of self-discovery that extends far beyond the mat. 5-4-3-2-1 methodology is in action in almost all sessions that Vaibhavi Haridas leads and some testimonials of actual students who have taken classes regularly are included in the next section.

In a world where yoga has become a commercialized trend, Ethnik Yoga stands as a bridge between ancient wisdom and contemporary life. It is an invitation to reconnect with the soul of yoga—to move, to breathe, and to awaken a deeper sense of awareness.

Ethnik Yoga Studio aims to host yoga retreats as well as teacher training programs in the future.

Learn more about Ethnik Yoga by visiting EthnikYoga.com.

Testimonials and Success Stories

The 5-4-3-2-1 Method has been a life-changing practice for many individuals, providing them with a pathway to improved physical health, mental clarity, and emotional balance. The unique structure of this method—combining asanas, sun salutations, meditation, chanting, and intention-setting—has resonated with people from all walks of life. In this chapter, we delve into real-life testimonials and success stories to illustrate the transformative power of this holistic approach.

The Power of Real Stories

When we hear about someone else's success, it inspires us to reflect on our own journey. These stories are more than anecdotes—they are proof that small, consistent changes can lead to significant results.

"I thoroughly enjoyed this session—it was both timely and deeply meaningful for my mind and body. The balance between informative content, physical workout, and meditation was beautifully maintained, creating a well-rounded experience. The session offered the perfect level of physical and mental relaxation, leaving me feeling rejuvenated. I particularly appreciated the inclusion of moon salutations, which are not as widely known; it was a wonderful reminder of these powerful asanas. Overall, it was an excellent session. Thank you for organizing it!"

"The session was amazing, Vai! Your voice for meditation was awesome, and the experience was superb. I felt new energy already to kickstart 2025!"

"I attended Vai's yoga classes (5:30 am batch), and it really helped me get into the routine to start my day nice and early. Her teaching techniques were amazing. Vai taught us something new every day that helped my body and mind in a great way. She's very knowledgeable, and I truly enjoyed attending her classes. I certainly recommend her! Thank you, Vai!"

"Vaibhavi has been very kind and understanding about individuals' abilities while teaching us, and she is very knowledgeable about the practices of yoga. By the end of the session, I felt that I could continue on my own with the simple asanas we learned (I understand that we could only touch upon a few things from this vast field) and keep myself fairly agile, active, and in good health. I got full satisfaction from her class."

"I absolutely love Vaibhavi's yoga classes! The pace is perfect, making it easy to follow along, and the live online sessions are a huge plus compared to recorded ones. She can see us in real-time, which means she can give corrections when needed. The class size is ideal, creating a comfortable, personalized experience. Yoga has always been close to my heart, but I never had enough motivation to commit to it until now. Thanks to my friend Vaibhavi for initiating these classes! I've already noticed improvements in my flexibility and strength, and I feel more confident and proud of my progress. Highly recommend!"

"As a yoga practitioner for a few years, I was looking for some deeper knowledge about the asanas as well as pranayama. Vai delivered! She is knowledgeable and always has a good plan for her classes, focusing on different aspects every week so that we truly learn and also enjoy. Her voice is soothing and supportive. Every class that I attended, I came away with learning and calmness. She is also able to motivate you to stay with your regular practice. Namaste. Many good wishes and 5 stars "

"Vaibhavi is excellent yoga guru. I love my weekly sessions. I always felt stronger with her guidance and weekly practice. As a teacher she is enthusiastic, calm and has wonderful voice. Her tailored sessions are great mix of strength, flow, deep breathing and relaxation. I always look forward for her Tuesday and Thursday sessions to regain my energy. Love yoga and best classes with Vaibhavi"

"Great sessions with detailed instructions. I was never into Yoga but Vaibhavi made me love Yoga. She ensures every person is following the instructions not just in in-person sessions but she does it very effectively virtually too. The app user experience is amazing too. Thanks Arva Yoga!"

"Arva Yoga has a Yoga lesson or a Yoga class for everyone. They have exercise and meditation sessions on weekday mornings, evenings, weekends. With their Yoga sessions, I was able to instill the necessary discipline in my routine with much needed daily exercises"

"Vaibhavi is very knowledgeable yoga teacher. I love all the sessions offered by her. The movement from one asana to another is very fluid and logical. My favorite asana is Moon Salutations. I look forward every Tuesday and Thursday morning for yoga sessions."

Key Themes from the Testimonials

1. Holistic Benefits:
   The 5-4-3-2-1 Method addresses physical, mental, and emotional well-being. From improved flexibility to enhanced focus, the method creates a well-rounded practice that resonates with diverse needs.

2. Personalized Guidance:
   Many participants praised the personalized attention they received during live sessions. Real-time feedback and adjustments help ensure that the practice is safe, effective, and tailored to individual abilities.

3. Simplicity and Accessibility:
   The method's simplicity makes it accessible to everyone, regardless of their experience level. By focusing on foundational practices, the program builds confidence and empowers participants to continue independently.

4. Consistency and Routine:
   Establishing a regular practice is a cornerstone of the 5-4-3-2-1 Method. Participants frequently noted how the method helped them develop a consistent routine, leading to long-term improvements in their overall well-being.

5. Community and Connection:
   The supportive environment fosters a sense of community among participants. Sharing progress, receiving encouragement, and connecting with like-minded individuals enhances the overall experience.

A Practice That Transforms Lives

The testimonials shared here are more than just words—they are powerful affirmations of how the 5-4-3-2-1 Method can transform lives. Whether it's starting the day with renewed energy, overcoming physical limitations, or finding inner peace through meditation, the method offers something for everyone. We would love to see your feedback on this particular methodology!

FREE RESOURCES

- Recorded yoga and meditation sessions
- Facebook Group for Support
- Free Live Yoga Sessions on Arva Yoga Platform
- Discounted price for Ethnik Yoga Classes where you can practice 5-4-3-2-1 Methodology Live via Zoom from the comfort of your home
- Exclusive invite to Retreats and Yoga workshops
- Discounted Yoga Teacher Training Courses
- Testimonials
- And much more!

Join the SHIVA Movement today! And be Inspired! Visit Ethnikyoga.com or email us at ethnikyoga@gmail.com for more information.

Namaste!

www.ingramcontent.com/pod-product-compliance
Lightning Source LLC
LaVergne TN
LVHW041119150826
845673LV00007B/2119

* 9 7 9 8 8 9 7 2 4 8 8 5 8 *